AUTOPATHY
HANDBOOK

D1739243

Autopathy Handbook

Enhancing Our Life Force

Holistic homeopathy without
homeopathic remedies, and beyond

Jiri Cehovsky

Those seeking help for any medical condition are advised to consult a qualified therapist, doctor or health professional. The information given in this book is solely intended for education and knowledge purpose and does not constitute medical advice or medical opinion.

Autopathy Handbook: Enhancing Our Life Force; Holistic homeopathy without homeopathic remedies, and beyond
© Jiri Cehovsky, 2019
All rights reserved
Translated by Voyen Koreis
Alternativa Ltd.
Zbraslavske namesti 461, 156 00 Prague
European Union
info@autopathy.com
www.autopathy.com
ISBN: 978-80-86936-52-9

Contents

Part Eight – The instructions for making an autopathic preparation

Introduction

Autopathy has developed from classical homeopathy. But its principles can be found also in the ancient wisdom of mankind; in Buddhist tradition, and in the Indian Upanishads. At the time of publishing this book, however, it is only sixteen years old as a method of facilitating a gradual return to health. It has been sixteen years of gathering experience and knowledge about how to help ourselves when our health is not in order, even if our problems have lasted for months, years or decades, and resisted conventional or unconventional attempts at curing. In such situations we could tune-up our out-of-tune selves to better receive the creative informational stream, which comes to us from the Universe and organizes our body and mind. This is called "prana" in yoga, the vital force in European healing tradition or in homeopathy, and "Qi" in Chinese traditional medicine. Such a harmonization in our practice has brought results – a revitalization, increased energy, better sense of wellbeing, and an improvement or even elimination of long-term health problems that are often considered incurable. Of this we – myself and my

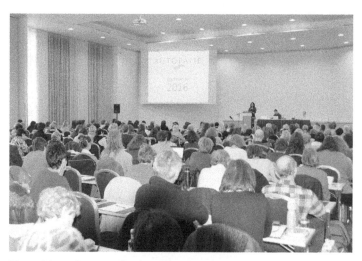

View of the audience at the 8th conference in 2016.

students – have become convinced. We often talk during our seminars and at our annual conferences, where people who use autopathy give accounts of their results and experiences. Many personal testimonies by users of this method, and the surprising results, can also be found in video recordings here: www. autopathy.com/testimonial or elsewhere on the Internet.

In this third book on autopathy I intend to give you organized and comprehensive information about what to do, and how to proceed towards the goal of improving eroded health and a sense of wellbeing and vitality – particularly when using autopathy on one's self, with family, or a circle of friends. These learnings could also be used in an autopathic consultancy service, should you run one, or intend to run one. However, even with the consultancy service, the client naturally and without a particular effort moves forward towards a scenario when he or she – with the help of a consultant – would become an expert in one's own prana, and thus one's own health. So that improvement should be interpreted by the signals that are being sent by our organism, and we can learn how to answer them. Autopathy is an art of handling the subtle pranic information that vitalizes man and maintains their harmony. The word "art" always includes an element of creativity, individuality, and overall insight. Consequently, it cannot be wholly fitted into strict rules and formulas, particularly when we work with such vast and mysterious spheres of man – such as his fine-matter (spiritual) dimension, which is responsible for what happens in the body and mind.

Autopathy is based on simple principles and it comes out of feelings, perceptions and observations of the person who is being treated, which are always our leading guidelines. Displays of our body and mind show our true state of health – our state of being and how it is tuned to creative intelligence coming from "above" – provided that we want to read these signs and are able to read them. Technical diagnostic devices, laboratory tests and similar things could be complementary, but not necessarily so. Autopathy brings us a health self-defense tool, such as we have never before had at our disposal. Furthermore, autopathy – the information method based on fine resonance – cannot cause harm to anyone.

In this book you will find a number of cases of treatment described. They show us that not only can negative states be turned around, but that the descent into more serious states – even when it might appear that the state of health is irrevocably been lost – can be reversed. However, these practical case examples show us the methods of treatment, and how the cure or a significant improvement of chronic problems were achieved, which had previously been proven to be incurable by other methods. I have described many cases from my practice of myself and my students in the previous books on autopathy: *Autopathy, A Homeopathic Journey to Harmony*, and particularly *Get Well with Autopathy*.

This book is meant to assemble the experiences gathered in sixteen years of autopathic practice; offering you the simplest orientation within the method, and providing answers to the most basic questions that the autopathic process of improving health could present you. It should be a household guide on the road to health, and is for anyone who is interested. Compared to my other books on autopathy, there are further cases described of returns to health, often from very disadvantageous positions of long-term, chronically ill people. Included are explanations of why I recommended particular parameters of treatment, with references to the rules of autopathy and how to apply them in practice, to gain results for yourselves or others. If you encounter a case similar to one in this book, you could proceed in similar way. In the book, a number of cases are also cited that some of my students presented at our ten annual conferences, or have published on the website www.autopathy.com. Without these practical and shared experiences, we could never accept, develop and successfully employ something so unbelievable in our world, as is autopathy.

For the best and most informed use of autopathy, naturally I recommend reading all three books and also the pages of www.autopathy.com.

The system of autopathy here is described chronologically, such as it happens in practice: How we begin, what we need, how we use it, how we evaluate the development and what we could do in certain situations or phases of the development.

Autopathy is not meant to replace any traditional, established, conventional or unconventional methods of improving one's health, and it could alternatively be added to any of these as a complementary method. It can also be, and often is, used as a self-contained method by people who have tried it, and come to like it. It is a holistic method capable of positively influencing the mind and body. It operates on a finer – but also more fundamental – organizational level, than most of the other known methods. There is a great level of freedom in its use. Freedom is the principal word. The aim is to get on the road towards liberation from being out-of-tune in body and mind; to lift oneself up away from disease and suffering, and towards harmony of a higher order. This way is feasible – many people have gone or are going through it, and have given accounts of the results they achieved at conferences, internet pages and forums, YouTube videos, seminars, articles, books, and elsewhere. Autopathic practice demonstrates to us, clearly and tangibly, that man is not only matter (which is literarily being hammered into our heads in school or by the mainstream media). Instead, above all, he has a fine-matter[1], spiritual dimension, on which our quality of life and feelings depend to a large degree. Autopathy is not only a method of treatment, but also a way of becoming aware of this dimension, which does not belong only to people, but also to plants and animals, which could also be helped by autopathy when applied at this level. Autopathy does not act on the physical body or mind directly, but solely by improving the connection of what we call the "organism" with our spiritual, fine-matter organizing common Source.

---

[1] The expression "fine-matter", which I often use, is adopted from Buddhist tradition, and its meaning roughly corresponds to the word "spiritual", while it more clearly expresses the fact that this fine level carries with it a prototype of material phenomena. See also The Dictionary of terms, p. 214.

If we work with information about any system of body and mind, and about its problems (such as diseases) there is only one possible use for these signals (symptoms of being out-of-tune). They show us the quality of its life force, prana, Qi, flowing from the fine (spiritual) sphere. We then work with this fine-matter – the most fundamental part of man – and through the fine-matter information transmitted by water, we aim to improve its reception and thus achieve better harmony of the chakras, body and mind. Terms such as "treatment" and "disease", have here only this one meaning. Autopathy treats our connection with the Source.

Nevertheless the autopathic principle is not specifically related to any philosophy or religion. Autopathy simply exists and should be viewed as a purely practical system of healing. Although I express certain philosophical opinions at some places in this book, they are not part of the method.

Autopathy has its rules, which can be easily learned. Some have been derived from practical knowledge of classical homeopathy, from which it originated sixteen years ago. However, the main body of knowledge has come by learning from many experiences with autopathic solutions of chronic states, gained not only in my own healing practice, but also in the practices of many of my students.

The volumes of water recommended to be used in dilutions are shown in liters. On page 235 there is a conversion table from liters to US fluid ounces and pints.

Part One

HOW TO DO IT

What do I need?

Autopathy brings harmonic fine information to our body and mind that rectify the damage caused by misinformation, such as so-called civilizational influences (which cause hundreds of negative impacts), and thus remove malfunction, disharmony, chaos and disease. It is an information method. This also means that the bigger your knowledge of the method, the larger your ability is to correctly regulate the individual parameters of autopathic effects and thus help yourself or other sufferers. From many people's accounts I know that on the basis of information gained from my previous books alone, great results can be achieved. However, there are other proven sources of information that people can use in healing.

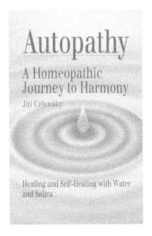

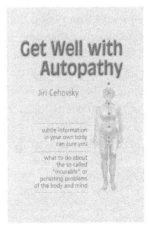

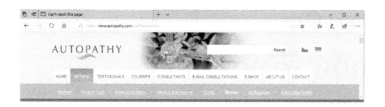

Amongst informational sources for autopathy, an important role is played online at www.autopathy.com, where fresh articles with descriptions of cures of chronically ill people are continuously being published, written either by people who have treated themselves, or by their consultants. Articles are there about the method; new findings that move the boundaries of our possibilities. Also published are news of techniques and strategies of managing cases, information about upcoming courses and conferences, and about everything else concerning autopathy. There are dozens of videos, in which people give their testimony of how they were helped by autopathy to overcome chronic and long-term illnesses. Many people who have been practicing our method have contributed to creating these pages, which are alive and evolving with each new contribution. The sum of their content is several times the size of this book. However, readers share one common experience. Whoever reads www.autopathy.com is welcomed into our particular domain. You can find contacts there to hundreds of consultants who have completed the cycle of instructional courses in autopathy, and those who are practicing it in different countries. *Whenever you read about these articles (quotations from them etc.) in this book, you can access their full versions putting their name or any keyword to the search bar on the first page of www. autopathy.com.* The same if you search for a name of illness, a kind of autopathic preparation or something else. There is a great material to study.

- **Autopathy bottle**

  An autopathy bottle **(AB)** is a tool for reliably making an autopathic preparation **(AP)**. It is produced in accordance with some special rules. The experiences and references found in this and other my books are related to the preparations made with it.

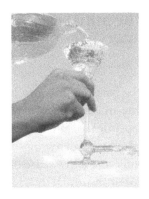

- You will also require spring water or filtered clean water, either from water mains (in which case we use a carbon filter), bottled spring water, or directly from a spring.
- When making a preparation from a fine-matter sample of a person – from the seventh chakra, or for making an AP for another person, a surgical mask is also needed.

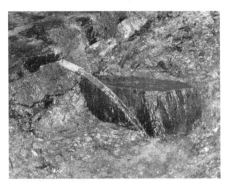
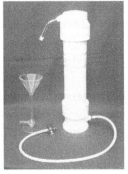

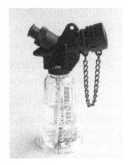

- Some kinds of autopathic preparations can also require a clean source of fire that does not smell or does not produce soot.

The initial examination or autopathic interview

The basis of our work begins by **thoroughly establishing the fine-matter's degree by being in an out-of-tune state** towards **reception of life force** by the person involved. This becomes evident through **symptoms**, i.e. disturbances in harmony, problems, and a lost sense of wellbeing.

For the initial interview we set aside about an hour, and we take notes and analyze the case (our own or somebody else's). No less than an hour, so that we do not rush our autopathic examination of the case. It will form the basis of further, perhaps even years' long activities. The follow-up interviews that happen afterwards will always be compared with the initial state and the state at previous follow-up consultations. Every one symptom separately and all its details.

Sit down comfortably with a notebook that you have dedicated to the case, or at the computer, where you have opened a new file (which you should always have backed-up).

You will **consider everything** that is troubling you. If you are interviewing someone else, you will ask the same question. **What are your problems?** Take notes of **all sources of suffering and negative feelings**, be it in the mind (such as sleeplessness, anxiety, fear, uncertainty, lack of concentration, hyperactivity, bad memory, anger…), or in the body (such as eczema, casual pain in gall bladder, menstrual pain, bleeding of gums while cleaning teeth, loss of hair, chest or stomach pains, painful joints, acne…). Write down each problem, symptom on a new line, and if writing on paper leave several lines empty between individual symptoms, so that you could, when you have completed the list of problems, return to it individually and update it with more details. Every person has a number of problems, *there is never only one.* Being out-of-tune prevents receiving the vital force, prana, which always causes a multitude of problems. One of them may have been the main reason for your decision to try autopathy, but we record them all. They all will be subjects of treatment, because the real subject of treatment is the state of being out-of-tune with the reception of creative and organizational life force. By tuning it up, we regain health and we force the source of disharmony or disease to retreat. With some people there might be only three problems, or "*symptoms of disharmony*", but with others there might be sixteen. If you happen to have on hand any diagnoses by doctors, specialized names of problems, test results, you can also write them down. *However, the most important thing to have on record is how these troubles are being perceived and observed by the person involved: this is the basis of properly monitoring a case.* The display of our feelings and perceptions is the most important and reliable guideline. We only treat one thing, the common cause of all negative feelings and disturbances of health, the disturbance in our reception of life force, otherwise bringing us perfect creative information and harmony. We always repair a malfunction in the fine-matter system of body and mind.

After we have written down all the problems, *the big ones as well as the small ones*, we can ask the following question: "*What else would you (or I) want to improve in your (or my) person?*" That is when problems, large or small, concerning for instance also our social functioning, relationships, professional ambitions, spiritual achievements, and such, could come forward. Even here we could, as has been found out, improve a lot with the help of autopathy. As counselors we should never try to lead any subject of treatment to saying more than he or she wanted to tell us, in order to help us with the examination. If we examine ourselves, we could naturally write down even those most secret sorrows, fears, traumas or wishes.

Afterwards we return to the noted problems (symptoms) we have taken and add **details** to each of them.

Localization – where exactly is the problem. 'The right knee, low left under the ribs, pectoral bone', etc.

Intensity – light, strong, terrible, unbearable, barely noticeable, etc.

Restrictions it brings with it – what does it affect. 'I cannot walk unaided, only with crutches or a stick, 9 miles in mountains and I can't go any farther,' etc.

Time fluctuation – time when the symptom appears, or when it gets worse. 'From time to time, constantly, once a week, twice a day, only at night, only at springtime,' etc.

Duration – from the first appearance of the problem till now. 'I have had it for thirty years, the past two years, three months, since yesterday,' etc.

Outside influences – external factors that influence, cause the problem to appear, or aggravate it – the type of weather, certain kinds of food, the temperature, staying at the seaside, working, etc.

History of health – here we record the more important points of bodily development from birth till the present, such as more serious or repeated problems, injuries, operations, long-lasting use of medical or recreational drugs, homeopathic remedies, etc.

Establishing and applying the three parameters of treatment

When we have gathered all the information, we begin to analyze it, in order to establish the **three individual parameters of autopathic tuning-up.** These are:

- ■ **The level of dilution, the potency of the AP.**
- ■ **The way of making the AP.**
- ■ **The period of application.**

What is the autopathic dilution or potency

We want to tune an out-of-tune organism to better receive fine creative information – life force, prana, Qi – and thus treat a malfunction, or rather an ailment or disease. To do this we have to raise the curing information to the state of fine matter, where our vital force will be employed. Information from one's own saliva or breath must be fined-up – so that its resonance is able to correct a disturbance in the subtle information system and thus the organism's malfunction.

Sixteen years of experience with autopathy means sixteen years of using the AB. The degrees of dilution are, as in homeopathy, called the **potency**. The higher the dilution, the higher the potency. The traditional term "potency" should not be taken literally, as it means "power". However, the healing effect is not generated by power, but by tuning-up the out-of-tune system, so it can once more receive the fine and perfect information from the Universe, and resonate with it and faithfully intertwine itself with it.

The ability to receive information, prana or vital force is at its strongest, nevertheless, when we use the degree of dilution that suits the best level of fine matter disharmony of the individual.

Too much water, a so-called "high potency", might sometimes have weak effects, as could potencies that are too low for an individual case. We therefore use the word "potency" (fining-up the information through dilution by water) out of piety, as it evolved historically from homeopathy, to which autopathy is closely related.

Working with the potency is the main art of autopathy. In autopathy, even very fine scaling in levels of an AP dilution are possible and sometimes necessary.

Determining the degree of dilution

Determining the amount of water that would in any particular case be poured through the autopathy bottle – or the degree of dilution, is the basic parameter with which we work. Should we decide arbitrarily or inappropriately on the degree of dilution – or fining up of information, the healing resonance might not be achieved. At best it could only be partial and imperfect, but in any case unable to properly tune-up the diseased organism. If the chosen amount of water is at least close to being correct, there might be a curing resonance. Individually, these degrees of fining up might vary, and we have some rules on how to do it.

The degree of dilution is to be determined individually for each case, taking into account the level of disharmony, disruption to its ability of receiving life force, and to harmoniously develop itself with it.

We find out the level of being out-of-tune from the depth of disharmony or disturbance that the system of body and mind has reached.

In simpler language: if there is a chronic disease of the liver, heart, or lungs, then the level of being out-of-tune is high and it means that the system's ability to organize its own self-defense is very low. Otherwise, the functional disturbance seen in the breakdown of such inner organs, which are so important to maintaining life, would not have happened.

On the other hand, if a healthy person sometimes catches a cold, which disappears within a week, or has a short fever that leaves no chronic, lasting problems, then there is a high level of harmony. The system of body and mind is still well organized, and it does not allow any disturbances, or any chaos or pathology to reach deep into the inner organs. It can defend itself successfully on the periphery, and it can quickly re-establish harmony that will continue. The highest level of being tuned-up to receiving life force is shown by the person having no diseases, even acute ones during seasonal flu outbreaks.

In this day and age we hardly ever meet people like this, though in the past centuries it was not such an unusual phenomenon. We have reports of people who have never been ill in their lives and who have died in an advanced age after a short bout of pneumonia or a similar acute disease, without a great deal of suffering, or even without any obvious pathological cause. They simply died of old age. They departed, having found out that they have fulfilled their mission in this life. For instance, the founder of homeopathy Dr Hahnemann (17551–1843) was healthy and kept working full time until the age of 88. In our polluted world of today, this hardly ever happens anymore.[1] People have long-term chronic diseases for many years before the end of their lives – and their resulting quality of life (including their sense of wellbeing) is low. Illnesses and health disturbances are the overall result of outer (environmental) and inner (karma) factors, which lead to disharmony in the organism, and the lowering of its ability to receive the creative information from the Universe.

The ability to resist diseases, create and maintain a harmoniously functioning system of body and mind – even under unfavorable conditions, and the ability to receive the fine information, is called vitality.

With a very high vitality (through organization and tuning-up), we reach a natural state without diseases; one we only seldom meet within today's chronically ill society. The good news, however, is that many people who were originally in a poor state of health, have nevertheless achieved it after the autopathic tune-up (particularly in young or middle age). The ideal goal of autopathy is to establish such a perfect state, and even though we might be aware in individual cases that perhaps we could not be able to do it, still our effort is directed to ideally reach it.

---

[1] Eurostat, the statistical authority of European Commission (government), showed that in 2013 and 2014 there is a shortening or stagnating average individual "healthy life expectancy" in many European Union member countries. In some of them, such as Germany, Belgium, Denmark, Holland, Austria, Switzerland, Finland, Portugal, Slovakia, this healthy life expectancy is already under sixty years of age, with Malta having the highest by far at seventy-four years. Having reached this age, the average woman begins to live in a state of permanent "disability" when help from other people is needed), and lives in this state for another twenty years (Germany, Holland, etc.. Males usually remain in this state for a shorter period, because on average they die several years earlier than women. http://ec.europa.eu/eurostat; Healthy life expectancy at birth.

High vitality people can cope with polluting and out-of-tune influences even on the periphery, and would not let them get deeper inside. People with high vitality are those who from time to time, but not often, get an acute fever, head cold, cough, rash, which they quickly overcome, and their good state of health continues. Or at worst they may only have a superficial chronic illness that does not restrict them.

Medium vitality is the state we encounter most often as healers. These are the people whose ability to maintain the state of harmony has gone out-of-tune to such an extent that it lets through various chronic symptoms, which not only persist, but begin to reach the inner organs that are important for life. They could manifest through serious disorders of digestion, such as ulcerous colitis or Crohn's disease, or strong rheumatic problems. Their energy levels are down, and they might suffer chronic fatigue syndrome, or insomnia. Tests might discover parasites or an increase in liver activity, thyroid gland, high level of sugar in blood, high blood pressure, etc. More prominent, also, can become states of anxiety, fears and depressions, arthritis, or strong migraines. Allergies might become more pronounced as well. *Essentially, the feeling of being healthy has disappeared altogether, or it is only there sporadically, and the restrictions caused by the disturbance in health might be seriously affecting the person's life. Nevertheless, the person's ability to maintain their social roles, to look after their family, go to work, etc., is still there.*

Low vitality means having in a state of being that is so out-of-tune towards receiving vital force that it enables the pathology (disharmony, fault, untidiness) to move deep into the inner and life-essential organs and systems, and threaten its existence. Signals of low vitality include a damaged heart, lungs, liver, kidneys, blood, upturned metabolism, malignity, or a strongly disturbed psyche. The problems that people with low vitality come to consultants with might be for instance an ischemic heart disease, bronchial asthma, chronic inflammation of kidneys, polycythemia and other faults in blood formation, multiple sclerosis, cancer, autism, and psychosis. People in this low vitality category frequent doctors' surgeries; they usually have had plenty of diagnoses, and have a long-term history of using chemical preparations. The feeling of wellbeing with these people of low vitality just is not there, and their overall state of being out-of-tune might even threaten their life.

The term *vitality* must not be confused with hyperactivity, workaholism, aggressive behavior, manic states or similar manifestations of increased activity. To us it exclusively means the organism's ability to maintain harmony and defend itself against disorganization, or a penetration of pathology inside the system of body and mind.

There is another criteria that determines the degree of vitality or ability to defend itself that we ascribe to a particular person: **their age**. The ability to maintain a healthy body and mind usually gets lower with higher age. In practice, it means that if we have in front of us a fifty-year-old lady and a child with exactly the same problem – eczema, for instance – we rate the lady as having medium vitality and the child as having high vitality. However, the age is a secondary criterion; a child with a serious inner disease – heart disease, malignity or liver disease – would always be of low vitality.

At the beginning of the autopathic treatment we judge the amount of water for the autopathic preparation (AP) made in autopathy bottle (AB) according to the vitality of the person being treated and we have three possibilities:

- With people of low vitality – 1.5 liters of water.
- With people of high vitality – 6 liters of water.
- With a person of neither high nor low vitality, but somewhere in between, it is medium vitality – 3 liters of water.

To determine the degree of vitality, details of the person's health history are also important. If there were some serious problems of inner organs in the past, be they latter improved by lifestyle, diet, medical treatment, etc., this leads us to decide to lower the degree of dilution, even though the current vitality might be higher. For instance, the current vitality, due to a serious change of lifestyle, might point to 3 liters, however, if the person had suffered a heart attack some years back – start with 1.5 liters. **With people over the age of sixty we always start with 1.5 liters.**

The initial choice of dilution – or potency – is important. Right at the beginning of treatment we want to find the autopathic preparation with the highest effectiveness. With a person of low vitality, 6 liters of dilution might have only a limited effect or none at all, while the result could be the same with person of high vitality and only 1 liter. Incorrect potency, however, cannot cause any damage. It is about **optimizing the effect**. We can even correct the potency latter by changing it after observing the further development of a person.

In summary: At the beginning of an autopathic tune-up we have only three possibilities: **1.5 liters (low vitality), 6 liters (high vitality), or 3 liters (medium vitality).** This is so with all preparations made of bodily information (such as breath or saliva), which are at the core of autopathic practice. **The exception is when preparation is made directly from prana**, the fine-matter information from the seventh chakra, where a different rule exists regarding choice of dilution (see page 74 – Prana – simple process of self-treatment).

Making an autopathic preparation

Autopathy bottle

An autopathic preparation (AP) is made in the autopathy bottle. It is normally made by the person who will use it, but it

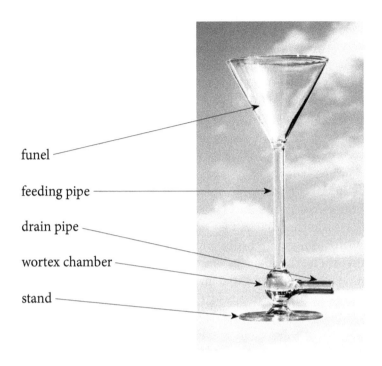

funel

feeding pipe

drain pipe

wortex chamber

stand

can also be done for someone else. Usually it is made in the bathroom, though making it in nature by a spring or water well is also appropriate. We have sixteen years of experience working with the autopathy bottle (AB). At the beginning we were tuning-up some ambiguities in the instructions for use, removing some imperfections, but very quickly we have arrived at the state where the instructions is well understood by its users, easy to follow, and enabling them to make preparations of a standard quality.

The AB is put in a plastic sleeve, which is zip-sealed. It can be found in a paper box, together with the instructions for making the AP (the standard are instructions for a preparation made from a person's breath). First of all, we read the instructions. We are aware that there are several other instructions, which vary in certain details. These are useful for specific states of being out-of-tune. It does not mean that in such cases the standard preparation described in the instructions would not work at all. It is about **optimization** of the process. Mostly we are facing serious chronic disorders, generally regarded as incurable, and anything other than optimized action would not be appropriate. All such instructions are included in this book (page 221). They can also be found on the site www.autopathy. com/instructions (see also the search engine at the first page) ready for printing, and each way of making preparation is also shown on video.

The AB is a glass tool, in which the standard preparation of the fine-matter substance happens. Inside, the body's information is subtilized. By elevating this information to the fine-matter sphere we make it possible, on the principle of resonance, to make the fine harmonious vibrations that organize our body and mind resound again, and return them, and thus gradually also the organism, to harmony – to health. Our bodily and spiritual system is always to a great degree tuned-up to our vital force, even when we have fallen ill. However, in such a case the tuning-up is no longer of a good quality, and we have to improve it. So, through better reception of vital information we can fix the problem. On the basis of this similarity in frequency (it is called "similarity" in homeopathy), the autopathic information from the organism is always related to its life force which has created the body and mind[2] and can help us to gradually tune it to better reception, and to make it possible for the fine creative energies – prana, life force, Qi – to sound again and be received in their original beauty and intensity. The fault can gradually disappear and natural harmony returns, even on the material level of bodily organs. This is not a theory; we have been observing it in practice.

You can read in detail how we proceed in making autopathic preparation (AP) in the instructions below, or you could also see it in video at www.autopathy.com/instructions.

---

[2]   In the fundamental work of homeopathy, The Organon of the Healing Art by S. Hahnemann it is written: "Man is ruled by the spiritual, vital force, which animates the physical body (the organism)…"

In our experience, so long as we adhere to the items in the Instructions, it is almost impossible to spoil making of the preparation. It is quite simple and takes, including the application, only a few minutes. By pouring through one liter we make the homeopathic potency of 40 C/2 liters, 80 C/4 liters, etc., in the AB.

Before our first preparation, we read the instructions, which we keep handy somewhere near the hand basin and check occasionally, to see that we have not missed anything. When we make the preparation for the third time and more, we will not need it any more – it is that simple.

The water

Water is able to carry the fine matter information, and it has been doing this in preparations (by dilution) of homeopathic remedies for over two hundred years. During the process of dilution and dynamization within the AB vortex chamber, water fines up the body's information, so that it can resonate with the fine vibrations of life force. Water forms 70%–80% of our body mass, and it is also the medium that connects the fine information sphere with the material world.

We set the flow rate of the water so that **the surface levels up with the edge**, *or slightly overflows it*. In such case a steady column of water forms, and the process of making the preparation is optimal. If the in-flow of water is less than the outflow, that would be a **mistake**, and the leveling of water in the funnel and subsequent water column would not form. In that instance the recommended potency *would not be made properly*. This could happen, for instance, when using a filter that allows only a slow flow of water. A stronger, even much stronger stream than the AB can take is okay, as the surplus water flows over the edge of the funnel.

When water bottles are being used, they will often need to be changed (as many bottles are no more than 2 liters in capacity). When changing bottles, the level of water in the AB drops down for an instant, but when more water is poured the surface in the funnel is restored. The changing of bottles should take only seconds, so the bottles to be used should be uncapped before you begin.

In countries where water in the mains is not being chemically treated (some towns in the USA, Germany, Switzerland, etc.), water directly from the mains can be used. Check the website of the local water supplier. Also suitable is water from a home system fed from your own non-chlorinated well. Some Internet sites also list the locations of natural water springs, can you can locate one near your home. There must be a pipe with the flowing water, under which we place the AB. If we use the spring often, even regularly, it would be useful having it cleaned at least once a year.

If we allow the water to overflow slightly or with the level surface forming near the edge, the AB lets through approximately 1 liter of water in 30 seconds.

We do not need to measure the water in any containers (in fact it is not allowed as any such vessel can spoil by its impurities in the preparation), but we look at a clock or timer (30 seconds = 1 Liter). The same applies if we use a carbon filter. If we attach it to the water mains, it would remove the chemical additives. Filtered water is good to use in autopathy, and this has been well verified in practice. Quality carbon filters can be bought online and in stores.

Removing the chlorine is important. Despite the warnings in the instructions, there have been instances where chlorinated water had been used, and the autopathic preparation did not work. Positive results from treatment occurred only after this mistake was rectified.

What to be careful about when making an autopathic pre preparation

Even though making an AP is simple, there are certain risks that need to be avoided.

**An AB should never be contaminated by bodily informa-
tion from another person.** For instance, it has happened that
a bottle arrived through the post, someone else from the family wanted to have look at it, and took it out of its sterile plastic
wrappings. By breathing on it from up close and maybe speaking, the bodily information of that person was transferred to
the inner surface of the AB in the form of microscopic droplets. In such a case, the contaminated bottle can no longer be
used by the target person, as it would not work. There would
be a mixture of information from two people. The resonance,
on principle of which the AP affects the life force, the prana,
cannot happen. For the same reason, the person who makes
the AP must be alone in the bathroom, and should make sure
that no one else would enter. Even if someone talked from an
open doorway, the droplets could be transferred by a distance
of several meters and ruin the preparation and the bottle, which
cannot be used then.

If we make the preparation for someone else, we need to
have a face mask covering the mouth and the nose, before we
even unwrap the bottle. We never touch the inside surface of
the funnel.

Similarly to the AB, the water could also become contaminated. For instance, if someone removes the chlorine from the
water mains using an open carbon filter vessel that was also
being used by the whole family for drinking, they could contaminate it by way of passing droplets. Such water could not
be used. Similarly, when someone fills water bottles for someone else from a forest spring. At the same time, his or her own
information is being transferred to the water by breathing or
talking. This would be a mistake. Yes, we can fill bottles from
the spring. We buy from a shop bottles with spring water and
use it with a face mask while making the AP for someone else.
Then we immediately close them, then take them to the well,
where we first put on the face mask, then fill up the bottles, and
close them – it is only after this that we can take off the mask.
A similar process can also be used in the case of having an os-
motic filter, which can have a slow rate of flow that would not

allow a level surface to form in the funnel of the AB. In this instance the water could be siphoned into bottles, which can then be used for making an AP.

The water needs to be pure H_2O as much as possible, with as little as possible of anything else to contaminate it. Common minerals that it contains are no problem. Somewhat higher content of some substances, such as calcium, magnesium, iron, nitrates, etc., do not negatively affect the quality of an AP. However, it is certainly not recommended for water to be "informed", to have any presumed healing quality, be it from the increased content of some minerals, or because of some healing effect of homeopathic information or similar. All this could reduce the effectiveness of the AP. The only subtle information that we want to have is content in the bodily or pranic information of the person being treated. It should otherwise be disturbed as little as possible. The water here is only a neutral transmission medium. However, light bacterial or other pollution that does not change the taste or color of water, for instance from wells or streams, usually does not cause problems. There will be more on this theme in Part Three, where we discuss faults we might encounter, including descriptions of cases where such problems occurred, were recognized, and removed. Such problems occurred only sporadically.

With boiled preparations, watch for the quality of the flame! Candles, lighters or similar sources of fire, which produce smell and soot, or are not designed to heating up, but only for firing up, **are not suitable**. Recommended instead are gas burners with a clean flame, either portable or stationary – there are plenty of them available. Gas burners for camping are also suitable, and if we use one we touch the small flame to the round vortex chamber with water in it.

A bottle can be used repeatedly with success for three months after the first use. From the preparation of homeopathic remedies it is known that glass has the ability to preserve potency. We call it the "memory of glass". From the first use we thus "imprint" our initial information into the AB; a week later there will be new information and also the one week old imprint; after that two old ones and one new, etc... The similarity to our present state is getting weaker and weaker. Our state changes constantly, and it is never the same a day later, let alone a week later. Therefore, the ability of the AB to resonate with our present state is slowly decreasing. We have noticed, and it has been debated at conferences, that approximately after **three months**, regardless of the number of uses, the similarity and with it the reactions to the application, begin to disappear. Occasionally this happens earlier, which we can easily detect and correct by changing the bottle earlier. In this book you will find several cases where this had happened (for instance, „The case arising questions", page 155). In the book *Get Well With Autopathy* I included a case from a conference, where a lady informed us of the unpleasant results of delaying a change of AB, and a relapse of a much improved Alzheimer's patient into the original state, which was overcome only by changing the bottles. However, I consider three months of use to be safe, and to be appropriate in an overwhelming majority of cases. Sometimes such a short period of treatment is sufficient for a long lasting improvement of a condition (see psoriasis, diabetes, blood pressure, p. 178).

Determining the best kind of preparation for your individual case

Presently there are six sets of instructions we use for making AP from physical information. For making AP from pranic information we have three instructions, which do not differ in the way of preparing, but do differ in the way they are applied to the organism and its chakra system.

It has turned out that some ways of making AP might be more effective than others in different states and situations, even though it might be possible for any of them to work to (some) degree – but not optimally. If our aim is to cure incurable diseases, nothing but the optimal way will do.

> **At the beginning of the autopathic treatment it is appropriate – with the exceptions stated later – to start with bodily information that was put through a boiling process.**

This is even more important when there is any inflammation in the body – chronic, acute, auto-immune, or any other.

1. Preparation from boiled breath (BB), instructions page 223.

At the beginning of the treatment this is the most commonly used method – it is almost universal. It is suitable in cases where auto-immune problems are prevailing, for instance when some organ or body part, etc., is being destroyed by one's own organism, its own "immune" system – auto-immune problems. At the beginning of the autopathic treatment it may be used by someone with a thyroid gland problem or similar hormonal imbalances, with faults in the inner organs, particularly the heart, and the whole circulatory system, including varicose veins. It is also applicable for people with viral infections, and in cases where tests have confirmed chlamydia pneumoniae, toxoplasmosis, or similar parasitic infections or respiratory problems. Similarly, where there is a chronic problem of an unknown origin, or a problem that doctors were not able to give diagnoses.

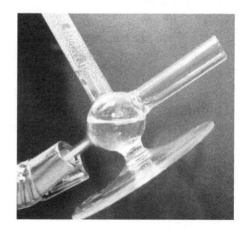

2. Preparation from saliva boiled (SB), instructions page 225.

This is the next type of preparation that is most often used at the beginning of an autopathic treatment. It comes into consideration as the prime choice in cases where the main problem has a yeast-related symptom, such as genital discharges, mycosis, digestive troubles, bloating and irregularities of bowel movements, hangnails, inflamed nail beds, white tongue in the morning, chronic fatigue syndrome, or cravings for sweets. If bacterial infections occur. Also eczemas, mollusca, acne and other problems where some puss is present. As well as all problems of the digestive system, from the gums, mouth and throat, through the bowels, and to the anus.

3. Joining the two previous methods: Saliva, breath, boiled (SBB)

Joining the saliva and breath in one preparation with boiling comes into consideration when the problems described in methods 1 and 2, both appear and we cannot tell which feels the worse.

Spit to the funnel, incline the AB, splash the saliva to the vortex chamber with water, then continue following instruction for the preparation from boiled breath.

In such cases we could also simply alternate between methods 1 and 2, for instance saliva one time, breath the next, using the same potency and the same bottle. This is suitable particularly with the lower potencies, under 6 liters.

4. Auto-nosode, instructions page 231.

Generally, if any substance comes out from any diseased organ freely and in a natural way that bears direct information of the given pathology, such information could be processed basically the same way as in making **the preparation from saliva with boiling**. This gives rise to an auto-nosode (a term

35

adopted from homeopathy) made from this substance, which can be more effective in treating this organ. This was used only exceptionally and always for a short period of time, sometimes only one-off, aimed rather at a specific physical symptom, and only in cases where other methods of making the preparation (from saliva, breath or prana) have not had any visible results. In our practice, for instance, we had a case where there was a festering discharge from fistula in the place where an open fracture of the arm was surgically treated. While the bones with metal supports were healing, the festering fistula did not. However, the next day after application of auto-nosode made from boiled and diluted pus, the fistula was healed, which the previously used autopathic preparations could not do. The planned surgery was cancelled. More details could be found in this article by Krystof Cehovsky "Autopathic preparation from pus – rescued at the last moment" (www.autopathy.com). **For finding any article on the website by its name, use the search engine the first page.**

In chronic cases, the use of stool has also been successful. It was applied for a limited time of a week or two, or only one application. It can be applied alternately in a chain of applications with another AP, in cases where the preparation made from saliva or breath did not have a full effect, using a low potency from 1 to 6 liters.

Also considered as an autonosode can be a preparation from the boiled urine of a person suffering from chronic inflammation of the urinary tract, or having a high uric acid level in the blood, gout, etc. I have even heard about the positive effect of boiled urine on diabetes.

5. Preparation from unboiled saliva (S), instructions page 229.

We dilute clean, fresh saliva in an AB in cases where cleaning had already been achieved through repeated applications of boiled preparations, usually using higher potencies than before.

Clean saliva as the first choice comes into consideration in cases of nursed infants, where it has been proved successful.

It can also be used after injuries and accidents of all kinds, including poisoning and such, as a first aid, *which is always at hand (see Korsakov's method of dilution*, page 135*)*, in addition to conventional first aid, which should naturally also to be used.

Alzheimer's disease, also known as "old age dementia", is an illness that affects more and more people these days, sometimes even well before reaching "senior years". Here, unboiled saliva is the first choice: we do not know why, but this way of making the preparation has had the best results.

People sometimes begin self-treatment with unboiled saliva (it was part of the standard instructions for use, included in the AB's box, before it was replaced by instructions for using the breath), which was often repeated in low potency of 1-3 liters. This has brought about some remarkable results. A cure was also achieved through the use of high potencies without boiling, applied on a one-time basis in the system "wait and watch" (also latter in this book). Nevertheless, the aim is always to **optimize** the effects, and currently it is thought that at the beginning of treatment, the SB or BB is more effective than saliva without boiling. It creates more space for use of an AP from unboiled saliva or rather breath, usually applied latter at a higher potency.

6. Preparation from unboiled breath (B), instructions page 227.

Developmentally this is newer, and in many cases it was proven to be more effective than saliva without boiling. It can be applied even in the highest potencies, after gradually increasing the amount of water. Sometimes it leads to the "ending" of the treatment by curing – it has happened that after high potencies (30–200 liters of water) from breath without boiling, a long period of health followed in many cases, without the necessity of more treatment. Most suitable is repeating the boiled breath or saliva in increasingly higher potencies, and then applying breath without boiling in a substantially increased potency, for instance twice to five times the previous one – and then "wait and watch" (the case "Lupus erythematodes", page 120). I have witnessed several times that its use resulted in the complete solution to the problems, lasting years (the case "Juvenile arthritis", page 187). Unboiled breath could also be used in similar situations instead of unboiled saliva following our latter experiences.

If the person's cooperation in the preparation of potency is unfeasible, the following way of getting fine information is possible:

A certain lady wanted to treat her dog and make a preparation from breath. It was nevertheless obvious that the sturdy dog will not allow any pipe be applied to his nostrils, and even if it did, it would be any good because of his restlessness. She did the following: She cooled the bottle in a plastic bag in the fridge for a few minutes (in winter you can put it out on the window), then using a face mask she brought the funnel of the AB to his nostrils when he was exhaling. The funnel grew dewy, and the dew was immediately washed with a small amount of water into the vortex chamber and diluted. The dog thus received the preparation from its breath, and the owner was happy with the progress. *In practice, a similar procedure could be applied in cases of **any person who cannot cooperate**, for instance being in state of coma, a sleeping child, and, of course, an animal.* The information enters the bottle and we can either dilute it downright, or boil it first. We have had some good results with this. Breath coming out of the mouth can also be used.

Application of a preparation made from information of the physical body: The water remaining in the vortex chamber after the process of dilution has ended, with the preparations described above, is dripped onto the space of the sixth chakra in the middle of forehead above the eyes, as is to be found in the instructions for use.

Chakras are fine matter energy centers. We can imagine them as to be spatial formations – like a cone, cornet or funnel – in the cases of chakras two to six horizontally penetrating the spine channel. The first and seventh chakras are orientated vertically in the axis of body, under the body and above the head. It is shown in the supplied image. Through this system the life force moves, entering through the seventh chakra from the higher fine matter sphere, and forms and nourishes the whole subordinate system of chakras.

The human body and its chakras, fine matter energy and information centers:

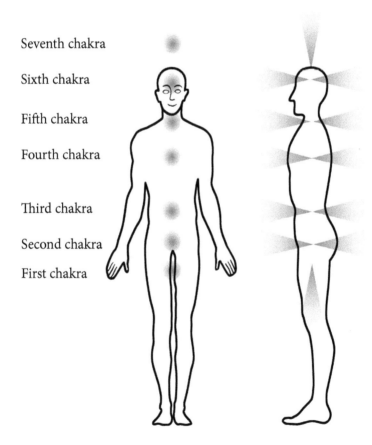

Seventh chakra

Sixth chakra

Fifth chakra

Fourth chakra

Third chakra

Second chakra

First chakra

The seventh center is 15–25cm/6–10" above the head, and the bodily chakras have centers in the skin's vicinity: the sixth chakra between the eyebrows, fifth chakra on the throat near the Adam's apple, fourth chakra on the chest – in line between the nipples in men, third chakra about 2cm/0.8" above the navel, second chakra above the pudental, while the first chakra is between the legs descending vertically. These are never the exact spots, but rather spatial areas.

7. Preparation from prana (P1 – P5), instructions pages 232, 234.

We can make autopathic preparations from the information of the seventh chakra. It is a round space the size of average watermelon situated 15–25cm/6–10" (in proportion to the person's height) above the head. I call it **preparation from prana**. The seventh chakra is the true center of an individual person. From here the human being materializes in our world by means of the lower chakras, as seen on the picture above. The seventh chakra is connected to even higher chakras, of an even finer substance, which become less and less personal – the highest chakra of all being the Source. As a dry theory this might sound interesting, but we were very surprised by the penetrating and sharp effect of the preparation on our feelings and the whole mental sphere. Many of those who made their reports at conferences have devoted them to this theme.

Preparation made of prana can be considered when the core of the problem, the main perceived suffering, is in the mind. *It might be for instance depression, fear, anxiety, strong worries even from ordinary situations, restlessness, strong inner tensions, insomnia, loss of memory, or there might even be serious mental illness. Belonging here might also be disturbances in social behavior, strong aggressiveness (for instance in children), autism, or a lack of concentration.* And other disharmonies that affect the mind in particular. Even though such a person might also have physical symptoms, making the preparation from prana is a first choice – it might improve or even cure also some physical symptoms present in a person whose main problem was perceived as being psychological.

Making the AP is always the same: We hold the water in the round vortex chamber near the bottom of the AB, 15–25cm/ 6–10" above the top of the head, in axis of the body, for about two minutes. The bottle is tilted, so that water does not pour out through the outlet. Afterwards we dilute it. We always wear the surgical mask, even before we take the bottle out of the wrapper, so that there would not be contamination from our own bodily information. The instructions on how to make preparations from prana vary, depending only on the method of applying the AP. Individual ways of application have evolved historically in the order of the number they bear.

Instructions Prana 1 (P1) – Apply a few drops onto the skin on the forehead, in the place of the sixth chakra.

Instructions Prana 2 (P2) page 232 – Drop onto the sixth chakra, and then go back again and inform the seventh chakra by holding for 30 seconds where the information was gained from, then hold the vortex chamber for 30 seconds tightly on the skin in place of the sixth chakra. To be used only when the source of problems is felt psychologically, while the physical body is relatively in order. Also when there is time or enough patience or some other reason, why not apply the AP to all chakras.

Instructions Prana 3 (P3) – Contactless application to chakras, in descending order from sixth to the first. This is effective when there are (besides psychological problems) also some physical problems in the parts of the body belonging to the lower chakras (the genitals, digestion, etc.). Application is essentially contactless: the water stays in the bottle while we hold the vortex chamber with the potency in the bottle tilted, so that the water cannot flow out, for half a minute by each chakra, beginning with the sixth, and ending with the first chakra. The first and seventh chakras are open vertically up and down; the other chakras take space horizontally in front and behind the body, in form of columns or tubes.

Instructions Prana 5 (P5) page 234 – The same as in P3, moving the potency from the sixth to the first chakra. However, after this we move upwards again to every chakra until the sixth, where we finish. *When using a new AB for the first time*, we can begin with the application to the seventh chakra and then continue to the sixth, fifth, etc… But in following repeated preparations with the same AB we usually start the application in the sixth chakra and do not return the potency to the seventh any more. We can try though if it gives us better feelings. With each chakra we hold for half a minute. Through such upward movement, the focus is brought back to the higher chakras. P5 has had the best results, and from all types of applications of preparation from prana I recommend it most often. Nevertheless, I often hear about good results with P1 from self-treating people. It showed us at the beginning how effective application made from prana could be. It is popular because of its simplicity and the speed of application. I was led towards applying the preparation made from Prana to all lower chakras by the insight that people might have some of the lower chakras blocked, perhaps the heart one. Then it would not let the vital information reach those chakras lower in hierarchy. Some problems of organs related to lower chakras thus could not be influenced. Application to all chakras and back again informs the whole system. Whereas Prana 2 has proven to be successful with prevailing and even severe mental problems related only to highest chakras, where there were no significant troubles on the physical level.

We have noticed that sometimes the influence of the preparation can be felt very strongly even at the moment of application. It could be experienced as the feeling of warmth or even of heat in the particular chakra, or as tinkling or prickling, streaming of water. However, this happens only in some cases and not always. Even when the immediate feeling is not there (usually it is not), the tuning could be successful.

The most reliable way of individually setting the degree of dilution and the interval of application with the preparations made of prana, is different from the preparation from the physical body. It is described in the Prana section – simple procedure – how to work individually with preparations from prana and be guided by one's own feelings, on page 74.

Instructions for all the ways of making AP that have been described above there are available at the end of this book. You can also find practical video demonstrations on www.autopathy.com.

Determining intervals between applications when beginning treatment

At the beginning of the treatment we nearly always repeat application of the AP at regular intervals.

We know that chronic (in other words, incurable, long-lasting) diseases have a natural tendency to keep getting worse. If we do not treat the condition in time, then the pathology will penetrate deeper inside. It will breach another line of defense, which could mean, for instance, that the skin might be cleared of the years lasting eczema, but instead the lungs might be attacked, giving rise to asthma. One's health and overall life enjoyment falls another level and limitations that the disease brings about are larger than ever before. The chronic disharmony after such a "cure" of the skin or other peripheral organ may affect the more important – for the person's life more meaningful sphere – inner organs. This can be deemed as a mark of deterioration in the overall chronic state, and of being out-of-tune with the reception of life force.

The criteria for how to apply the autopathic preparation is the speed of deterioration of chronic state of health up to that time. The frequency of application depends on how fast the chronic out-of-tune state of body and/or mind deteriorates.

In the treatment of long lasting chronic problems, the standard interval between applications is once a week.

Nevertheless, if the speed of deterioration of the overall chronic state of disharmony is high, we apply the preparation more often.

In situations when there is a sharp deterioration, or a direct threat, we apply once or even more times a day (typically as an auxiliary method to conventional treatment).

More frequent applications of more than once a week could also be subject to the feelings of the person being treated. For instance, when positive results (increased energy, reduced pain, better sleep, etc.) caused by the preparation disappear after a few hours or days, a frequency shorter than a week needs to be undertaken. If the **speed of deterioration of a chronic state is only slow** (for instance, the migraines, joint or other problems, even though they might be strong at times, are about the same frequency and intensity as last year), we might apply the AP less often, for instance only once in 10 or 14 days. Such a prolonged interval could also be used with potencies of 12 or more liters, which have been reached by the gradual increase in the amount of water.

In my consulting practice, I had originally been recommending **intervals of applications of one week**, but usually I added a caveat: **or more often in case of problems.** The qualification is there so that if any crisis came (at the beginning it is more likely to come than with the subsequent treatment), I can apply the preparation more often, perhaps once a day, still in the same potency. After that we can return to the original interval of once a week. Among such crises could be a temporary, short-term worsening of a symptom, or some acute event – for instance a one-day fever or cough. In this context, I stipulate that treatment and harmonization – the tuning-up of chronic problems – is usually a gradual process. It must be remembered that at the beginning of the treatment we certainly

44

are not healthy, and the inertia of the condition's pathology persists.

Usually, people at the beginning, and often during the autopathic tuning-up, visit their doctor, just as they did previously, which is only natural. **Autopathy and self-help aren't substitutions for medical treatment.** Doctors usually treat with material substances that have direct effect on the material body, while autopathy exclusively stimulates the fine-matter (vital force, prana, Qi), which from the materialistic point of view is immaterial. As it has turned out, these approaches, active on two entirely different levels of human beings, do not quarrel, and can even complement each other. The fine-matter part of man, however, is more important than the physical part from our point of view. It is the primary part, because it has created the body and mind and is its life.

Sometimes it is possible to **undervalue the potency with regard to the vitality of the person being treated, and pour less water into the bottle, but apply more often, perhaps daily.** For example: A lady is of a medium vitality, which would indicate 3 liters, once a week. Instead of starting on this, she would have 1.5 liters daily, perhaps for 14 days, and only after that move onto 3 liters once a week. Even with such a tactic, the consultants have achieved great results, when the most suitable potency was preceded by a preparatory phase with a lower one.

A particular way of application is a system called **"wait and watch"**. It consists of just one application and no more; it comes into consideration roughly from the potency of 30 liters onwards. The higher potencies sometimes have the ability to tune-up the organism for a prolonged period, and after only one application. The observation of the treatment's development consist of asking ourselves if it is in line with Hering's Laws (page 50), but more about this system in later chapters. We usually arrive to "wait and watch" in advanced stages of the autopathic tune-up. Use of a one-off application at the beginning of the autopathic process of tuning-up is possible, and I have described a number of such cases in the previous two books. However, there is more emphasis on observation of the person's development. Practice has shown us that repeating regularly at the beginning has its irreplaceable advantages, particularly with self-help.

The reason for our meticulous analysis and selection of the most suitable method of making and potency of the autopathic preparation and interval of application is the **optimization** of effect. We cannot say that the three parameters of treatment set up somewhat differently, less correctly or randomly, would not do something for the person, if the making of the AP is correct. But in cases of chronic problems, when we aim at complete elimination of an otherwise irresolvable and incurable problem, then only the optimal effect is desirable. Sixteen years of experience, shared with a large number of people (for instance at ten annual conferences), have handed to us valuable tools enabling us to make the treatment as intensive, short, and the best possible, for any given person.

The end of the first consultation (self-consultation)

Take the AB, and on its wrapper we write down the **three individually chosen parameters – 1) the amount of water, 2) the way of making, 3) the interval of application**. If we have a consulting practice, we change the instructions that came with the box (instructions about preparation from breath) for the one that we have selected and printed for the person being treated. They all appear as PDF files on the pages of www.autopathy.com/instructions and also in this book on the page 221 onward. Onto the box we write for instance: 3 liters, breath boiled, 1× weekly till follow-up interview.

If we recommended the Prana system – basic procedure, we follow the instructions on page 232, 234, which we can also print from www.autopathy.com/instructions.

We recommend the treated person to record any obvious changes in their condition.

Regardless of whether we treat ourselves, a friend, family member, client, or patient, **it is appropriate that the person being treated records any changes in their condition with the date of occurrence**, and also parameters of the AP application. With self-treatment we could write this into our file or notebook – where we have recorded the initial examination, and later the follow-up interviews. The feelings and states of body and mind of any person fluctuate. In times of illness it might be conspicuous, but even with healthy people these feelings change – they are different in the morning compared to the evening, depending on changing situations, weather, events, etc. That does not need to be closely observed. Records, with the date of occurrence and disappearance, need only be the feelings or changes that defy ordinary fluctuations of the condition.

Development after beginning the autopathic process

System of follow-up examinations

In cases of chronic illness that have been long-lasting problems, the organism generally needs some time – weeks, often – for drawing in energy, before the first noticeable marks of reaction appear. If we treat another person, **we set the date of first follow-up examination at five or six weeks** after beginning the treatment. If anything happens that stands out compared to the ordinary daily fluctuating state, the person concerned should make note of it in their notebook or special computer file. Writing notes on a computer might be impractical, as it could be difficult to read them during a consultation. Some people bring these notes on a flash drive, but many people don't accept other people's flash drives, because of the danger of viruses. Computers can also catch diseases, and autopathy does not work on those (don't even try it!). However, with self-treatment we can safely use our own computer. Otherwise, a paper notebook is generally better, as no virus or hard drive crash could spoil it.

The system of follow-up examinations is very simple. During the initial interview we let the treated person speak out and try not to interrupt them, and generally try to keep distant in our approach.

During follow-up interviews we ask questions. We look at the initial record and simply compare **each symptom, each problem, all its details, with the current state of this symptom or problem.** We leave nothing out, and we follow-up on any details recorded during the initial examination.

We do not skip anything; we follow the initial record from the first line down. And perhaps we find out that the first recorded problem has not changed at all, the second symptom on record is 50% better, the third has gone away, the forth has gotten slightly worse, the fifth is the same, etc. We document it all in the follow-up examinations record. We also note things such as the person's overall feelings. **Sense of life** is something that you would rarely be asked about during a medical examination, yet it is what forms our sense of existence, our basic frame of mind. Improving our feeling of life is the main motivation for everything we do. Whether choosing our occupation, partner, place to go to holidays, treatment, buying new things like clothes or cars: anything at all. We always expect that it would improve our life sense, which usually does not happen, or only for a while. And, surprisingly, people often state that the lasting improvement of their feeling of life is the first mark of overall improvement, the feeling of goodness, which sometimes comes even before any gradual improvement in condition of the afflicted organs would have been noticed. The inner part of man, the soul – the awareness, all that is closest to the life force, prana, comes into tune first. And we know it, we can feel it, our body feels it, and people around us feel it. In some cases this is what happens. In others, the sense of wellbeing grows gradually, with fluctuations: the road is never simple, and a lot depends on the initial hidden state, on the person's karma. An important question during the follow-up examination is: "**How do you feel?**" And the answer, after some reasonable time of autopathic tuning-up has passed often is: "good", even if some problems persist. If the answer is "bad", we have to think about changing some of the parameters in our treatment – even if physically there have been some improvements.

The follow-ups that come later would have a larger interval, perhaps once every two or three months. The period between applications also usually gets longer. With some people, in time (after years of autopathic treatment) the follow-up examinations happen only when they think about it, maybe after several months, even years. **When we continue follow-ups, we compare the state of every one symptom recorded during the previous follow-up, with its present condition. However, for the sake of orientation we keep returning to the original state recorded in the first interview, even after years.**

When the treatment slows down, we take the time to carefully study all the previous examinations. Thus we can find out, for instance, which potency or which way of preparation brought the best results, and return to it. Or we might discover that a certain kind of method of preparation has not been tried yet, though it could be useful. From the detailed records of follow-ups we can better see if our case has been developing in line with Hering's Laws, or if the positive development has stopped and does not continue… With self-treatment we naturally pay attention to our state often concurrently, even after years. Important here is the realization that it is not desirable to constantly change the parameters of treatment because of short-term fluctuations of our own feelings. With these fluctuations it is important to teach ourselves to a wait a day, two, or a week, before we move onto any justified changes. You can read more about the specifics of self-treatment on page 199 and, naturally, in the context of the entire book.

In assessing the sometimes complex holistic development of the condition we have the help of Hering's Laws.

Hering's Laws of correct development in holistic treatment

The body and mind during the process of an autopathic tune-up react in a peculiar way. First of all, usually the parts of our organism closest to our fine-matter sphere – the mind, improve first. The improvements then move to the parts of the body in accordance to the known anatomical hierarchy, first being the most important ones – heart, liver, kidneys, blood… This wave-like movement of healing from the fine-matter sphere towards peripheral areas of personality, mind, and body, was described in the classical homeopathy, and was named "Hering's Laws of Cure". Dr Constantine Hering was an American homeopath of the 19th century. He described this system of treatment on the basis of correctly selected and holistically effective homeopathic remedies, and tuning-up the system of body and mind towards the state of health. Following the advancement of harmonization, tuning-up – in accordance to Hering's Laws – gives us the ability to correctly react to a condition's various stages of development, which could sometimes appear at first sight to be confusing. When we add the criteria of Hering's Laws, all becomes much clearer.

The human organism is a dynamic system and nothing in it remains unchangeable and ever-lasting, in good health or in illness. Essentially it can move only in two directions, upwards or downwards; towards the state of health or deeper into the state of disease. Towards more harmony, happiness and orderliness; or contrarily away towards disharmony, suffering and destruction. Whenever the development moves downwards – towards growing disaster, which is given by the nature of our world in which we live – the disharmony afflicts more and more important organs. The model of development might appear thus:

*The first of Hering's Law states that individual symptoms (problems) in a case are to be solved in the direction "**from within outward**".*

When the holistic tuning-up of life force lifts the organism up, the first to be cured are the most important and most threatening problems on the inside: in mind, in heart, in liver, etc. Only then towards those problems on the outside like on the skin, nails or hair. **The most important, the most threatening or limiting, therefore the "innermost" problem has to be resolved first**, while problems on the fringes can stagnate or fluctuate out of inertia in a persisting out-of-tune state, until the healing wave reaches them, which always emanates from the life force, prana, towards the outer sphere of the body.

There exists a "healing intelligence" – our Higher Self, our fine-matter pattern – that when you have become better attuned to it, would decide on its own what truly is most important for you. It sets itself to work accordingly on those things that are most serious, that limit you the most in your natural health potential. What we usually call intelligence, is only part of what contains intelligence of the Higher Self, which has created the entire body and which keeps it alive. The intellect we obtain from schooling and our cultural environment is built in it. But it is only a filtration, screened out in addition by the out-of-tune state of our body and mind, unable to receive the perfect information from the higher sphere. By tuning-up our higher sphere (it is indeed ours, not something exterior and distant), everything moves into order, always depending on the degree of the individual's state of disharmony here, on the physical level. It happens in reliance to our karma, the hidden state of our mind and body. We have noticed that some people – despite of their advanced age, a high out-of-tune state of their inner organs, and an overall decrepitude – move towards health faster than others, who might not even suffer from a serious pathology. But they have to overcome a great number of obstacles and eliminate many impurities that have built up in their body and mind. This is where differences in people's karma come into the equitation.

In this regard, people are not the same, and we do not have the ability or the tools to enable us to judge at the beginning of treatment what sort of karmic endowment we might expect to encounter in a case. The karma of a person can put obstacles in their treatment. It can stop it, even thwart it. A materialist, at a certain moment when there is an obvious improvement, could abandon the treatment, to save his set of values, his vision of the world and of himself. For the same karmic reasons, strengthening or salvation of a belief system, people are sometimes capable of sacrificing lives (theirs or somebody else's). Karma might cause a person to not find out about autopathy's existence, even though there could be many people around them who have had great results with autopathy. He is not attuned to such information; in his karmic development he simply has not arrived to it. In my experience, people who choose autopathy on their own generally are not too badly off in the area of karma...

Autopathy, however, is not a philosophy, but a practical tool for improvement – we make our autopathic preparation and we record the results. They usually come, in various measures, regardless of whether the person in question "believes" or "does not believe". Autopathic preparations have even helped babies, whose mothers made them while they slept, and did not even found out about the treatment. Even dogs, horses, cats, and also plants, generally alive but unaware organisms, have reacted to it very well. All life has its roots in the Source, and it is connected to it through prana. Anything living can fall ill, when its reception to harmonious fine-matter information is weakened and out-of-tune.

Therefore – if we see an autopathic treatment set that is in accordance to the three parameters (degree of dilution, way of making, and period of application of the AP), and the problems are withdrawing in accordance with Hering's Laws, **from within outward** (for instance, the first to improve is heavy insomnia, liver tests progress next, the urinary bladder after that, and the skin last), we would not change the autopathic set-up and follow it to achieve more positive developments and results that it would in all probability keep bringing about, until the state of tuning-up of the organism does not change.

Nevertheless, if a previously well-adjusted treatment with regular applications begins to eventually break down – it has not been the same lately, the case is no longer heading upwards – or **the previously cured symptoms reappear**, *this means that the development of symptoms, the pathology, begins to* **"move inside"**. *In other words, there is a* **relapse, or a decline in pathology**. *In this case the current degree of dilution has used up its possibilities, and the* **first thing we do is we increase the degree of dilution**. *Thus we could once more resurrect the proper way of development "from within outward".*

> **When a previously successful and regularly applied potency is exhausted and ceases to improve, or even when previously solved problems reappear, we always increase the dilution. First usually by 1.5 liters.**

Most often, particularly in the early period of treatment, we increase by one bottle of water, or 1.5 liters. Things might then move in the right direction. If not, we increase by a further 1.5 liters.

The same applies when the reaction after the early applications is not too obvious or discernible. Again, we increase the amount of water. However, a great deal depends on correctly following the case holistically, and careful matching of all parameters – all of them, not just a selected one – with the initial state. In one case, it repeatedly happened that a lady in the process of treatment forgot about already removed long-term problems, and instead of them at the follow-up interview she now accentuated the current, even superficial problem, so that it might have appeared that the treatment did not do anything to her. I had to remind her of her initial state, *comparing all the original symptoms with their current state.* In that instance she originally suffered from strong anxiety, insomnia and tiredness. In her current case there was no longer anxiety, she obviously has more energy, and her sleep was getting longer. It was then that she suddenly realized that a lot has changed (the case "Nothing has changed", page 150). People have a remarkable ability to quickly forget about the cured chronic problems, as if they never happened, and focus on their current state. Also, I have always explained to people that if the process follows Hering's Laws, from inside out, the deep-seated problems that are most endangering and strongly affect the life, improve first, while on the periphery the pathology persists, waiting for its turn. Therefore it would not be proper to change anything in the setup of autopathy. If it moves in the right direction, improvements in some physical problems in this process are not to be left out; they will also be cured, but later. Much of how the case develops, if it moves up or down, in line with Hering's Laws or against them, we find out from the records in the notebook of the treated person. Quality of these concurrent recordings is important for the correct process of autopathy.

The hierarchy of symptoms in the organism, which the holistic treatment follows, is as follows:

The deepest seated are problems of mind; those connected with a serious inability of assessing reality – delusions, psychosis.

Also extreme emotional disturbances, such as chronic fear or anxiety.

On the next level is the overall state of the whole organism, chronic fatigue, very bad sleep and its consequences.

Curing of physical symptoms usually keeps in line with the known anatomical hierarchy. First the heart, next the liver, nervous system, kidneys, lungs, organs of blood formation, and other inner organs essential for life, such as the endocrinal system, digestive system, etc.

At the very end of the bodily hierarchy are the skin, nails, hair, whatever is on the surface, on the organism's periphery.

Our life force begins the tuning-up process of mind and body with symptoms that are the deepest seated (on the top of our list), and ends with those that are at the periphery. The process is automatic, we never think of trying to target only one item on our list with autopathy and leaving out the others. *We never treat separate diseases, but always the whole person, from the seventh to the first chakra.* Diseases and health problems happen when our overall state of being is out-of-tune with the reception of the life force that creates the organism. When the system can no longer accept it due to being severely out-of-tune, it dies; if it accepts it partially, it is diseased; if it is well tuned, it is healthy.

The development of a diseased organism before autopathy usually moves against Hering's Laws; the problems move from outside, in. This is a natural state of decay, towards being out-of-tune, towards disharmony, to greater suffering, and chronic illnesses. First it defends itself on the surface, later the more and more important parts and functions are being attacked. The defense weakens, and gradually retreats inward, into the inner bulwarks. Like a siege of a medieval castle, where the enemy breached one circle of defense after another, until the capture of the lord of the castle, who lived in the innermost tower. The siege begins in an early age, as we have shown, through colds, rashes, followed by coughs and throat infections in puberty. In adolescence there comes asthma; the problems move deeper and deeper into the organism, and they are getting more dangerous, and depression or heart disease could follow... Autopathy might turn this development around.

In the process of conducting an autopathic treatment, it could happen that the **set parameters of treatment have been exhausted,** and unhappily developments turn towards the "inside". They no longer bring about the movement from "within outward". **They need to be changed.** For instance: The patient's insomnia has gone, then their sore knee recovered; this state lasted for two months with the same setting of the three parameters. But lately, the knee begins to be felt again and the sleep is not quite as good as it was recently, even though it is still better than before the treatment began. All is improved when compared with the initial state, but the development, rather than moving upwards towards less suffering and removing of pathology from inside out, is beginning to move in the opposite direction. Even the sleep is disturbed again – the inner portion of the person, belonging to the mind. *The development is against Hering's Law – the disharmony once more moves inside, instead of being pushed outside.* Even though we continue applying AP, the development is not good. The potency currently used has given us whatever it could, and it cannot do more. After such a realization we have to react by **increasing the amount of water used in the process of dilution, usually by 1.5 liters.** The development might again move upwards: The sleep improves, the knee no longer hurts, in the direction "from within outward". If the development still defies Hering's Law, we increase it again by 1.5 liters. If the case continues then still moving towards a state of disharmony and moving **from outside in,** or the overall sense of wellbeing is getting worse, **we consider change in the method of making the preparation,** which is another measure that we have on standby.

To be comprehensive, there are two more of Hering's Laws we must cover, but which are not as important, and have been derived from the first one already described. A case may not necessarily be developing strictly in accordance to them.

The symptoms are being cured in the reverse order of their appearance. If we have a long-lasting eczema, and insomnia that lasts only for six weeks, then the first to be cured would be the insomnia, followed by the eczema. Acute problems also belong here – because if a fever came today, while the insomnia has been there for some time, and the eczema even longer, first cured with the AP would be the acute fever (often within twenty-four hours, as we will learn later), then after a time the insomnia, and after a longer time still, the eczema. It is always holistically influencing the central problem, this always being the out-of-tune state of the organism towards the reception of life-force. *The longer the symptoms have lasted, the longer they have to wait their turn.*

With cases when the pathology is spread throughout the whole organism, for instance when the eczema covers the entire surface of body, or with polyarthritis, where many joints are sore, **the problems are usually cured in the direction from up to down**. Thus we have noticed that the eczema first disappears in the hair, then in the face, the chin, the low neck, and lastly at the ends of hands and legs. The same could happen with back pain; first to be cured is the neck area, then the chest, and lastly the lower back. Nevertheless, exceptions do happen.

To these known three classical laws of holistic healing, we add the fourth, which I would rate the second in importance. **The symptoms are being cured in order of importance**. Anatomical hierarchy is only one possibility. More important, however, might be the hierarchy of inner priorities of the person being treated. Sometimes it happens that first cured was something that caused a high social and psychological limitation, even though from the anatomical point of view it was not anything of inner importance. It could have been a sore leg that prevented social functioning of a particular lady (the "Case of Good Karma", page 102).

Symptoms in reverse order

Sometimes, for a while – a minute, an hour, a day, etc. – there might be some old, perhaps even completely forgotten, usually superficial problems that reappear for a short time. They could be psychological in nature – some old fear or dream from childhood, perhaps. The same can be true in the physical area – a small rash, a quick joint pain, a couple of days with a sore throat, etc. The way that a person descended into the more serious pathology is being followed upwards, and a reminder of some states is being met. Not all of them, by any means. They do not reach the intensity of the original problem, and nowhere near the same duration. They are always superficial displays, in reality the pathology is being forced to the organism's periphery by the life force.

These old symptoms, I call them symptoms in reverse order, signal to us that we are on an upward path. They are usually a sign of detoxification. From these kinds of signs we read that we are moving in the right direction, towards the state of overall better health. If an appearance and disappearance happens to be noticed, we are reaching the previous, better levels of existence, which were ours before we fell ill. And we move farther, higher and higher, as the three parameters of autopathy have been correctly set up. **I mention this, *even though in the large majority of cases, no such old symptoms are being noticed.*** Still, it is better to know about this possibility, in case they might appear briefly, and in line with Hering's Laws, meaning that the deeper seated problems were improved already. The classic American author of holistic homeopathy, J. T. Kent, writes: "… the ignorant do not desire their old outward symptoms to be brought back even when it is known as the only possible form of cure. (Lectures on Homeopathic Philosophy)"

The healing crises

Sometimes it happens that before a long-term chronic problem begins to disappear, it becomes slightly more perceptible for a short time, rather than directly improving. Naturally, it can happen only in accordance to Hering's Laws. For example: an aggressive child, who also has eczema. The mother is at her wit's end from the boy's aggressiveness; he has problems at school, he is greatly restless and constantly attacks others. During the autopathic treatment, the inexplicable aggressiveness improved first, then the eczema got deeper red (the healing crisis), but was less itchy, and in a few days began to disappear. Because the mother, despite the worsening state of the eczema, could see that the child is calmer than before, the worsening of the eczema did not concern her (the healing wave had moved from "within outward"), and soon could see it disappear.

If the healing crisis comes at all, then it is only short, and in order of the symptoms' hierarchy. *It is mild, it comes rarely, similarly as an old symptom in reverse. A healing crisis never occurs, and this can also be said about the symptom in reverse, in cases of severe diseases – particularly of the important organs.* In classical homeopathy, where these principals of holistic treatment were first described, we talk about **healing intelligence**. Treatments of the mind and body are better and better attuned to the information from the "Higher Self", which is connected to the Universal Source. This higher sphere is much more intelligent than an ordinary mind in any person, or the "reason" cultivated by school and culture. It has created the healthy body and mind, and it strives to maintain it. It knows what is best and good for us. The disease (a fault) happened because the reception of creative information was disrupted by disharmony of body and mind. The treatment restores its pouring of wisdom of the higher sphere into the bodily organs and mind.

Fluctuation of state

The development of the human organism and its feelings over time is never a straightforward one, be it in health or illness. We always have some emotional or physical fluctuations, and states of illness are usually larger and more conspicuous than healthy ones. It is this way due to daily or yearly cycles, food, stress, activity, rest, variances in quality of living environment, etc. We feel differently in the morning and in the evening. This fact has to be taken into account while following the autopathic development. The fluctuations in a normal (healthy) state should not cross the boundaries of "normality", which of course are subject to conventions and are changeable, which is quite natural. A practical recognition of these fluctuations in autopathy leads us to never comparing the treatment of chronic diseases with only today and yesterday, or morning with evening. We always think in terms of longer time spans, weeks or months, when we can clearly recognize that these fluctuations happen on a different and generally higher level than before. While short-term observation usually does not give us enough distance or perspective, which are **important for possible adjustments to the three parameters of treatment**. *If we had to react to every short-term fluctuation by changing one or all of the three parameters of treatment, we would not get far.* Let's remember this is particularly true in the case of self-treatment, when we do not have the benefit of distance from our feelings, which is the advantage of attending a consultation practice.[3] Therefore it is sometimes advantageous, even in self-treatment, to visit a trained consultant in moments of uncertainty, so that we might gain a second, objective opinion from an emotionally unbiased party.

At any stage of an autopathic tune-up, it is always possible to consult about the condition's state with a medical doctor, because **autopathy "is not a substitution for medical and**

---

[3]   You can find contact details for autopathic consultants at www.autopathy. com.

certified health services", as is stated even in all the instructions for making an AP.

How to keep follow-up examination accounts

Whether we treat ourselves or visit a consultant, we keep a notebook or a well backed-up computer file from the very beginning, where we record all changes in the condition **that defy their ordinary fluctuations**. This does not mean increased self-vigilance. However, when anything comes about that is an unusual or an out of the ordinary feeling, we write it down together with the date of occurrence as well as the departure of the feeling, manifestation, or symptom. It could be a slight headache, which normally is not there: "It appeared on the 3rd of May in the morning, and was gone on the 3rd of May at noon." But we do not record the pains we feel daily and which we want to cure. In such case, the recording could be something like this: "The last two day my headaches were not strong." Or: "Last week I only had the headache three times." Recently a gentleman phoned me, who has been self-treating back pains with the book *Get Well With Autopathy*. He said: "I've been doing this for 14 days, and recently I had increased the boiled breath preparation to 4.5 liters, twice a week. For the last two days I have known that it works. My spine, which gave me chronic problems for years is still hurting, but the last two nights, for the first time in years, I have slept throughout the night, whereas before the pain would have woken me up several times a night." Therefore, his recording should be "2x slept all night". He also noted that it follows Hering's Laws. First the mind reacted, the sleep, before the physical organs could improve. And what about the feeling of life? That was suddenly much better. I told him that while the setup of three parameters works well, and bring about improvements, nothing should be changed, and **he should continue in his self-treatment with the same setup of three parameters, so long as there are improvements**. Only if there was a stagnation for a longish time, or if the development had even changed direction and started to go down, against Hering's Laws – if the disharmony began to move deeper into organism, and the already cured problems returned (such as insomnia) – then dilution should be increased by 1.5 liters. If he had recorded nothing, in a few days we would get used to sleeping throughout the night, and he might easily be asking if autopathy did anything for him. Our experience has been that the unpleasant things, such as long-term insomnia, are those people tend to forget about quickly.

These records help us to re-construct the long-term development. Five or six weeks after the follow-up interview, we return to these notes and evaluate the progress in detail. We compare every recorded symptom and its details (intensity, timing, localization, the level of limitations, etc.) against the state at the time of the follow-up.

We act the same way during the follow-ups (or self-conducted follow-ups) that come later. We might also compare the results of laboratory and other medical tests that preceded autopathy and their development during the autopathic treatment. We can check that it was indeed the laboratory blood tests that showed first the signs of improvement, even before they were felt subjectively. **With self-treatment, we should be careful about not doing follow-ups every day, and not deducing hastily that changes in the three parameters are required from a short term development. We always allow up to several weeks to pass with a certain setup that we have decided upon, and only after that we should evaluate the development and perhaps alter one of the three parameters.**

In such cases, we normally change the potency first, usually by 1.5 liters. And if we have already reached higher potencies, then perhaps by a larger amount of liters.

Usually, we wait impatiently for something to begin to happen to our problem. This could occur right from the word go, but it could also take days, weeks, even months. **As a rule, the longer we have had a particular problem, the longer it has to wait for its turn to come.** There is also the influence of karma. We cannot say that all people react the same way to treatment of the same problem. Three people of the same age and same level of disease might react like this: With the first person the disease goes away after two days, with the second after a year, and with the third perhaps not at all (it may be that he has something to learn from it).

When we have set-up the *individually suitable* three parameters correctly, the results come kind of automatically, and they might even happen without us noticing. Therefore having correctly recorded notes is necessary. For instance, a certain lady was waiting to see what happened to the problems with the joints of her lower limbs. She attended a follow-up interview, and with disappointment she said: "That knee is still hurting." Her expression was skeptical. I looked into her records and asked her: "And is the right hip joint still hurting, as it did a month and a half ago?" The lady was surprised. "No, I completely forgot about that." "And does the knee still hurt so much that you have to use a stick even for short walks?" "No, in fact, I don't use the stick anymore." And thus, due to the recordings, we can both see that things have been moving in the right direction. The lady even remembered that the pains in her joints had originally begun in the knee, and later expanded to the hip. Therefore, the development is in accordance to Hering's Law: "The problems disappear in the reverse order of their appearance." The parameters of autopathy had been correctly set up; nothing needs to be changed, because they still affect the development.

People have the remarkable ability of forgetting about old chronic problems they had, if these become things of the past. It is also supported by the fact that to them the disappearance of "incurable" chronic problems is a brand new experience, and sometimes they cannot even believe it happened. A good recording that was done by the person being treated, or by the consultant, is therefore important. In the case just stated, we can also note that pain of joints is being cured "from up to down", which is the third of Hering's Laws: the symptoms appearing in the body (joints, eczemas, back pains, etc.) are first being cured on the upside, where they are the closest to the

63

individual fine-matter center of the person, the seventh chakra. From there the healing wave moves downwards.

During follow-ups, people often immediately identify the beginning of obvious improvements, of which they are fully aware, and express their thanks. This occurs particularly if they had started with a strong suffering, with a limiting chronic pathology, where the difference might have been noticeable not only to them, but also to those around them. On the other side, paradoxically, stand the more difficult – and for the consultants more demanding – cases of relatively healthy people. They may want to change their personality to gain more effectiveness in (for instance, economical) dealings, assertiveness, better performance and similar traits based on competitiveness in today's ruthless society, which however might not be in tune with the universal laws of harmony. Yes, such people can become more successful, we have seen it many times, but sometimes they must overcome within themselves the negative sides of their personality, which they used to think as being something positive – pride, hatred, etc. Autopathy could be useful even here, but the road is not a straightforward one, and it might not be so easy as the person in question imagined, despite otherwise being "quite healthy".

A technical problem could arise easily when treating a family member, a partner, friend, etc., whom you see often, and not because of autopathy. It might happen on the part of the treated person, that when we meet at the door, remarks are made like "Nothing's happening", or "It's still quite fine", or "That hand's still hurting". From this we cannot read anything at all about the person's condition. Treatment, the tuning-up that we seek, is always holistic, and it includes the whole of the mind and body, without fail. *Casual references should not be accepted. It is proper to let a few weeks pass, and then take half an hour together with the person concerned, solely for the sake of an autopathic follow-up examination, and to sit down in peace and* **compare each and other symptom from the past with the present state.** *Ask yourself the question: does the overall development follow Hering's Laws?* And usually, you would both see that much has been improved, so that the three correctly set parameters do not need to be changed. Or, with the help of the treated person's notes, you find that the improvements were there up until the previous week, but now the person involved is in a relapse. They are again falling into the previously overcome pathology, because the repeated applications of three liters have exhausted themselves and it is necessary to move to four and a half liters, to restore the positive results. Or it might come out that it would be advisable, perhaps because of a change in the symptoms, to change the method of making the preparation, maybe from boiled breath to information from the seventh chakra.

With self-treatment we use the same approach – every now and again we do a detailed follow-up of our out-of-tune symptoms, one after another, comparing even the details that we have recorded during the first examination. For example, a certain food no longer causes headaches; however, the headache still occasionally appears. The pollen season this time did not bring about itchy eyes, though the sneezing came again... Indoors, the tips of my fingers no longer freeze. By using such details (modalities, as they are called in homeopathy), and their comparisons, we may recognize an interesting development that shows if we have selected our three parameters correctly; or not, if no significant changes have come. Significant changes of course might be happening right from the beginning: sometimes people feel immediate and noticeable relief even within the first hours, days, or weeks.

The modalities then are not so important, but their details could provide indications to us of whether we are on the way up, or not. For instance, reappearance of a negative modality, which had previously been removed, could be the organism's early signal of a relapse, which could then be arrested by a change in one of the parameters of treatment.

Working with the potency

We know already that when the curing reaction that previously happened is stagnating for a time, or when it disappears, as our first reaction we increase the amount of water. Usually this brings about a stronger effect and the case moves again towards improved health. *The fact that a well selected potency in time loses its effectiveness is quite normal.* We must then work on an even finer level, to get further holistic developments. *Sometimes it happens that we increase the level of dilution too fast due to our impatience*, without waiting long enough to see if the given potency brings about a gradual progress. Or, if we do see progress, we want it to be much bigger and faster. Something has already improved, but that is not enough to us, so rather than repeating the same potency, which could have brought about a gradual progress, we increase and increase again. However, instead of further improvements we are met with a worsening condition in comparison to the lower potency. **In our impatience, we have leaped over the optimal level of dilution. Then, after examining the records of the previous development, we return to the dilution that worked best in bringing about positive changes**. The improvements will most likely come back. We keep repeating this dilution that brought us the gradual improvements, and move the case towards a cure. If we reduce by 1 to 4 liters, we can do so in the same bottle. But if it was by more, then the solution turned out to be taking up a new one, because the memory of glass could burden the new lower dilution with the old, more highly diluted information.

In the more advanced phase of autopathic harmonization we increase the amount of water whenever the development stagnates for a longer period. With the potencies below 20 liters we increase by 1.5 liters. **With the potencies over 20 liters, we increase by 3 liters, and with potencies over 30 liters we usually add 10 liters. With potencies over 30 liters we can leave the regular applications, and move onto the one-off applications, according to the rule of "wait and watch" (page 70),**

and step in only at the right time, particularly if we suspect there could be a relapse.

Changing the way of making AP

When none of the symptoms (of imperfection, disharmony) in our case for a long time (weeks) shows any positive improvements, or any positive movements towards more comfort and harmony, and we have already twice tried to increase the potency – with a gap of at least two weeks between applications, then we begin to think about *changing the way of making the AP*.

For example, we began with boiled breath and some things have improved (such as pains in joints), but a gynecological yeast problem persists. Not even increasing the amount of water by 1.5 liters brought about any changes, or only insignificant ones. This is the time to move to boiled saliva, which works better particularly with yeast related problems, and continue with the same potency as before. Nevertheless, after a time, when we have eliminated the yeast, we may realize that under the influence of some stressful event, our ability to fall quickly into sleep has become worse. In such case, we first increase the potency by 1.5 liters, and if that does not help, we move onto preparation made from prana (P2 or P5), which works directly on psychological problems. **When changing the way of making an AP to prana, we always start with 1.5 liters, according to the section "Prana – a simple method of self-treatment", regardless of how far we have previously been with number of liters while using information from the physical body.**

Changing and combining various methods of making preparations from bodily information

If we are not quite sure whether the appropriate beginning of an autopathic treatment is with the SB or BB method, we could simply keep changing them, one after the other, in the same potency and in the same bottle (Crohn's disease, page 116).

We could also do BB and a week later SB, and see which makes us feel better. If there is a significant difference, we could then move onto the method that has better results, and leave aside the other method ("Self-treatment – choosing the best way of making a preparation according to feelings", page 87).

If in the same case we see yeast (SB), and auto-immune (BB) problems, or vascular (BB), as well as digestive (SB) problems, we could simply make saliva and breath into one preparation with boiling. Cases, pages. 99, 126, 138, 150.

Alternating AP from prana and bodily information

Particularly in cases of severely out-of-tune individuals, it is possible to treat from two ends. You can add energy and improve the connection with the higher sphere with the preparation made of prana, and alternate this with diluted bodily information prepared with boiling. Generally we could use this approach if we want to have as much effect as possible: From above, the information of the seventh chakra, from below through the body's information. For instance, when there is a severe and threatening bodily pathology, usually strongly limiting the level of psychological wellbeing, then two separate ABs are needed. We recommend in all cases to begin with 1.5 liters in both preparations, repeating for a time in a regular interval; or often in urgent cases, and alternating methods, for instance **SBB in the morning, Prana 5 in the evening**. Alternatively, one day this, the other day that, or one week this, the other week that. A longer interval, such as one week, is suitable when there has already been improvement through autopathic treatment. Later we can increase the potency in accordance with the parameters of the case's development, the feelings and observations, and always repeat the same potency for a time. See case "Cancer, allergy, high blood pressure, sore knee BB, SBB, P5", page 99.

It is also possible to evaluate the parameters that determine the level of dilution separately for an AP from prana and for boiled bodily information, particularly when we have the time to observe the development and feelings after each individual application. This happens mainly after the preparation from prana, where the improvements in mind can appear soon or immediately, for instance with the interval of one week (the case "A lady and her boss", page 98). The degree of dilution of an alternatively applied AP can then differ (the case "Alternating SBB and P5", page 126). In time, however, we often get at leveling of potency, which may eventually be the same.

Preventative import of repeating AP

After a time, with regular applications the individual symptoms are gradually removed, and the person concerned no longer has any significant displays of being out-of-tune. If, however, the initial problems were significant and strongly limiting – such as bronchial asthma, a malfunction in the thyroid gland, autoimmune malfunction of liver, depression, etc. – then in such cases it is good to extend the interval, perhaps to one month, while continuing to apply the same potency that successfully helped to remove the problems. Or, in time increasing it and prolonging the interval. In our experience, when people have felt to be cured, and even tests have confirmed it, they did not continue with autopathy. They thought this was the end of it. Health is normal, isn't it? To their displeasure, after a year or two, the already cured pathology came back.

But there is logic in this. Unless these people changed their regular routine, which sometimes happens spontaneously after autopathy (food, movement, avoidance of toxic influences, perhaps even a change of environment, etc.), the conditions for another bout of the illness are still there. If we do not resist it by stimulation, through continuous tuning-up of prana (the life force), the pathology could gain the upper hand once more. If the problems return, it is necessary to begin treatment again, usually with the same potency and the same method of preparation as used immediately before the cure. *However, regular applications of potency in a longer interval (once every 14 days, or a month) helps to keep healthy and prevents relapse.* I have described several such cases in the book *Get Well With Autopathy*, 6th edition (the case of bronchial asthma; the case of autoimmune hepatitis).

Deferred application of AP

If we have reached the stage when symptoms and problems have slowly gone away, we could in time move from the usual weekly application onto 10, or even 14 days. Then we observe and see whether the last used application still improves and moves the case onwards, without returning to problems that were already overcome. If things are still improving – more sense of wellbeing as well as lesser pathological symptoms of mind and body – we may defer the next application and prolong the interval. Perhaps, to once a fortnight, later to three weeks. At the same time, we usually increase the amount of water. With the higher potencies, particularly 12 and more liters, the interval could be up to a month.

Wait and watch

In the course of time we might get into a situation when we do not apply the preparation for a long time. **We only observe the development and are ready to step in with applying AP whenever it is necessary**.

I have even had cases when it was not necessary for up to eight years after the last application, when a chronic problem such as an eczema, that was completely cured, had begun to reappear in a small way. At the same time, the lady in question did not have the usual influenza, or any other illnesses she had been suffering before autopathy. She was completely healthy.

One application in the same potency that preceded the cure was enough to make the reappearing eczema – only on the back of her hand (not on the whole body, as it was eight years earlier) – quickly disappear. **"Wait and watch" is the system of vigilance over the development, and recording any possible changes, while no AP is being applied,** *up to the point when there is a relapse (in line with Hering's Laws, the pathology begins to move "inwards", the development ceases to move in direction "from within outward").* Things might be improving for a longish or even long period. This wait and see period gives us a relatively easy task of when to step in with another application. This is because during the time many people usually were healthy – perhaps with only light, sporadic and superficial symptoms of detoxification, for instance fighting against an aggressive environment (typical head cold, etc.), which disappear quickly on their own. Nevertheless, when symptoms in the direction of outside-in appear, against Hering's Law, they are usually indications of a returning pathology (eczema, though a small one in comparison to the original state, headaches, painful ovaries, etc.), and it is then necessary to apply AP. We reapply the same AP that caused this long-term change, and keep the same three parameters. Usually one application was enough to solve a returning problem, which could have happened in a month's time, in three weeks, or in eight years. The change to the "wait and watch" system is usually preceded by a gradual increase in potency, with regard to the development of the symptoms always substantiated. If we move onto this system too soon, we return to the repeated applications of AP. See page 142, "The case full of mistakes".

I even have clients, whom I have met casually several years later, and who appear to still be fine, without using autopathy in between.

While observing the holistic development, we do not forget that nothing is static in the human body or mind, and that there are constant changes and variations. An important thing to note is that those variations do not exceed the level that, in feelings, as well as in medical tests, is considered to be beyond the boundary of pathology. *If that happens, and there is a relapse, we return to the potency and the method of preparation that had previously led to the problem's removal. If that no longer works, we increase the potency.* That can be applied once – if the problems go away and the state of health returns, we once again move to the "wait and watch" method. We keep records and make sure that the development is moving in the right direction "from within outward", in line with Hering's Laws of holistic treatment (the case "Switch to one-off application and the "wait and watch" system – the case of a child's eczema", page 112). In the "wait and watch" phase, we repeat even when we have a mere suspicion that it might be needed. In a case of a "premature" application of the same potency, which had previously brought about an improvement, we do not spoil anything.

This system is particularly useful with self-treatment, where we can follow our feelings in detail and react readily, if needed. In consulting practice it is necessary to explain in detail to the client the whole process, including Hering's Laws, because in the role of self-treatment and independent decision making is higher than in the system of regular applications. As far as my clientele goes, most of them have gone through courses of autopathy; some have had experience with self-treatment after reading the book, before they came to see me. Some cases were highly successful ones, when through consultation with me people wanted affirmation of their way of treatment, or simply to have a chat with me to tell me their – to some of them rather surprising – impressions of the development after an AP. Therefore most of my clients have the necessary knowledge for this method of observing their cases.

The common aim of autopathy is tuning-up the organism to the level of health and harmony, so that there is no need to apply any AP, simply because it is not needed. From this point of view, the system of one application and then "wait and watch" is the ultimate aim of autopathy. We move to this phase most often from when we reach potencies of 30 liters or higher, though in some cases the potencies are lower.

72

One-off application at the beginning of autopathic treatment

In the previous two books on autopathy – Autopathy: *A Homeopathic Journey to Harmony* and *Get Well With Autopathy*, I described cases when from the very beginning of tuning-up I recommended a certain well-chosen potency, and then we followed the development in line with the system of "wait and watch". Positive development sometimes lasted for a number of months, or even years. Then I found out that in some cases this method has its limits, and that repeated applications worked better with some of them. Later, I recommended to more people the method of repeating AP, because I found out its larger effectiveness. Naturally, the notion of changing to the "wait and watch" system is possible, but only after an improvement to the overall condition. Therefore, my recommendation nearly always is in the first stage of treatment: repeat at regular intervals. However, even now I mention this possibility of a one-off application at the beginning of treatment. It is suitable to people of high, or at least medium vitality, and unsuitable to those who have low vitality, who are over fifty years of age or who take regularly medicine, or who are exposed to outside, irritating influences that currently keep growing in amounts and intensity. As of fourteen years ago, times in respect to this were more friendly, for instance with regard to microwave radiation in the environment. Nevertheless, it does not have to be only the so-called civilizational technological impacts. Hardly anyone these days gives much attention to cosmic factors, the relatively fast weakening of electromagnetic field of the Earth, increased amount of cosmic rays that fall onto our planet, the changes in the Sun's activities, movement of the Sun around the center of the galaxy, penetration of the heliosphere through variously dense interstellar plasma, etc. And there are also changes in the fine-matter sphere. The transition to the new era, the Age of Aquarius (the New Age, the Golden Age – regardless of how we call it), and probably also a global shift in the mankind's karma, the on-going destruction of outdated models and notions, particularly the materialistic ones, which are trying to hang on by power control and losing credibility in people's minds… Fortunately, there are not only the negative influences that are getting stronger, it is also autopathy. The fine-matter sphere is always superior to the material one, so long as we are able to receive well its information, which is where autopathy helps.

Prana – a simple method of self-treatment, setting-up intervals and potency of AP made from the seventh chakra

Determining the degree of dilution "according to vitality" at the beginning of autopathic treatment is solely relevant to an AP made of bodily information. **The proper system of assessment for individual potencies and intervals with an AP made of information from the seventh chakra, Prana 5 or Prana 2**, are described in my article on Autopathy.com, and later also added to the 6th edition of *Get Well With Autopathy*. Many have been using it successfully. The system is simple; it is based on **careful observation of one's feelings, mainly in the area of the mind,** and adjusting the level of dilution of AP accordingly. No one could know your own feelings as well as yourself. It is really self-treatment, even though a consultant might be useful here. I base it on the experience that a preparation made of prana is capable of quickly and sometimes distinctively changing the psychological and energetic state, including the "life sense". But only if we find the specific level of dilution, the one that is "ours".

In all cases we start with 1.5 liters of water poured through the autopathy bottle, following the Prana 5 or Prana 2 instructions (pages 232, 234), and observe what it does, particularly to the mind. If within three days this level of dilution makes no significant change in our feelings, we add another 1.5 liters of water. If that does not bring about any changes in our feelings, on the fourth day we add another 1.5 liters. And so on. The aim of this relatively quick succession of applications and increases of water amount is to observe one's own feelings and find the fine-matter level that is "ours". We must find the level that best resonates with the individual, and that can reveal itself through *an obvious and undoubtedly positive change of feelings.* **It may be a change towards larger psychological comfort,** *such as a moderation of tension and stress, more energy, lesser emotional reaction in ordinarily stressful situations, more rest, a better mood, improved sleep, a greater sense of wellbeing, etc.* Singularly, it may even raise anger, a sense of unbridled energy, which in a few hours could change into positive feelings. Individually, the level of dilution might differ. We do not skip any of the levels while increasing them, so that we do not miss the one that is "ours". At the beginning of our autopathic movement it might be somewhere between 1.5 liters and 12 liters, regardless of vitality or age. I saw only one exception where it happened after 22 liters.

When we have found the level of dilution that within three days causes a positive movement in feelings, we repeat it regularly at an interval of once a week. *However, we apply more often if there is a decline of effectiveness in a time shorter than a week, for instance after three days. Or within five hours.*

If there is not a positive reaction by the time you reach 12 liters, it is appropriate to think of other methods of making preparation from bodily information, such as the breath without boiling, in a higher potency.

The same potency that had caused the positive change may deepen and strengthen its effect through repeated applications, and gradually solve problems, without further increases. **If we begin to relapse with repeated applications of the same level of dilution; or if we see that the effectiveness of the AP has diminished; or if the previously improved or cured problems return; or there is long-term stagnation, we always increase the amount of water in the AP by 1.5 liters.** The increase in the amount of water could restore the reaction. We can then stay on the same level of dilution even for a long time, while monitoring our feelings and repeating regularly once a week, or even more often, if the positive effects of the previous application do not last.

If the AP becomes less effective, or ceases to deepen its effect and keep positive change, we increase the amount of water – always by 1.5 liters.

If we are happy with the state we have reached – particularly if we have already reached the level of dilution of 12 or more liters, we could try to move to the system of **"wait and watch"**. This means we stop regularly applying an AP, and watch the development while it continues satisfactorily, if there are no signs of a slump in psychology or even a suspicion that it might be on cards. If that change occurs, without a delay we return to the potency that preceded and caused a positive reaction. For an illustration of how such a development might proceed, I include "The case of chronic fear, increasing potency P5 and final transition to Prana 5 D 74 liters", page 190, and "The case full of mistakes", page 142.

While looking for our optimal potency – or the level of dilution – sometimes the mistake is made when there happens to be an improvement after a certain number of liters (such as "I was in unusually good mood", or "I slept so much better"), but impatience pushes such a person farther to higher dilutions, which brings no improvements and even loses the previous gains. I had a case of a woman around forty years old, who after going through the course had begun to make P5, correctly from 1.5 liters. She had immediately felt a great improvement psychologically, lightness and relief. But she had said to herself: "If one bottle of water does this, if I use two I'll have these good feelings twice over". This did not happen; the effect was actually somewhat lesser. She attacked with three bottles, and was in the same not-so-good condition as before commencing autopathy. She came to see me and I had recommended her to return to 1.5 liters – immediately there was a relief. Only after about four months of weekly applications was it appropriate to increase to 3 liters to keep the good condition. It was a case of jumping over the optimal potency. The remedy is simple: return to the lower level of dilution that had brought about a positive change, and stay with it. In time other problems can be improved, the changes will deepen, and perhaps even reflect themselves on the physical organs. Increasing the amount of water should come at the right time, when the effect of the currently used potency begins to lessen.

To make the AP from prana, we use a thus far unused AB; there must not be (in its glass) information from the physical body, which is also averted by our wearing face mask. To make an AP from physical information in an AB that was previously used for "prana", is possible, the other way it is not.

If we gain a significant improvement of mental comfort, moderation of emotions, etc., it may happen, as it has done, that the physical symptoms follow (in line with Hering's Laws). Thus we had seen, after prana of low potency, alopecia (loss of hair in a young woman) disappear, also infertility (the case of Iva Marcantonio: "The message from London: A problem of conceiving a baby", Autopathy.com).

Or, after a high potency P5 treatment, fever in a child was gone within a few hours – the case of Fever, page 135.

I would like to stress here that even though I regard the making of AP from prana to be an important contribution to the method, it is more of a specialty, though very reliable after we find the right potency. The largest part of my practice remains to be making AP from breath with boiling or without boiling, and from saliva with boiling and without boiling. I also use all other methods and procedures described in this book.

Part Two

THE CASES

Having broadly left behind the theory of autopathy, which is not derived from speculation but from practice, we can now look how it all works in reality. We will look at some cases from my consultancy. The general rule is that each case is different, with its individual mix of feelings and problems. Even if the diagnosis is the same, the picture of neither the disease nor the way of treatment are ever the same. There are, however, rules of holistic treatment (particularly in classical homeopathy), and specific rules of autopathy, derived from experience gathered during practicing autopathy. If we apply them correctly, we could cure "incurable" diseases, and not only that, it can open up an as yet unknown stream of happiness and strength that changes not only ourselves, but even the surrounding world into a more friendly space to live in.

It was the cases, my own and those of others, that taught us how to go about it. If you have a similar case in front of you, you can proceed along a similar line, while at least adhering to the same rules that I stipulate in my commentaries to the cases.

A somewhat miraculous case, BB

A lady, over sixty years of age. When I ask what her problems are, she says she has bronchial asthma; she uses a spray even after a short walk. She also suffers from continuous headaches, which she has had for thirteen years, since she hit her head in a fall. She feels tingling in her right hand, somewhat lesser in the left; it is horrible and she is supposed to have a carpal tunnel operation. Sometimes the nape of her neck gets frozen and she cannot move her head. Her knees and hips are painful, and it gets worse when moving; when resting she does not feel it much. Her sleep is bad; she wakes up by 3am and usually cannot sleep any longer. She has a slight heart arrhythmia; sometimes she feels a tingle near her heart. She often has heartburn. Her back is very itchy; sometimes her elbow joints itch as well. She often feels restless, as if something in her was having a fight. She is treating a diseased thyroid gland and she takes a substitutionary hormonal preparation. She has light diabetes, near the high norm, and she keeps no particular diet.

Health history: In childhood she had repetitive tonsillitis, her tonsils were removed. She had infectious hepatitis. Six years ago Chlamydia pneumoniae and orrealia were found in her, and she took antibiotics. She said that she had decided to try autopathy after she saw how much it helped one of her friends, who had "improved unbelievably" after her treatment.

I recommended breath with boiling: **BB, 1.5 liters of water, every second day for 14 days. After this 2 liters of water every third day, until we held a follow-up interview.** I set the follow-up to occur in two months. Meanwhile, she was asked to take notes about any changes in her condition.

- *Why breath with boiling? The main problem was in the breathing tract, so information from there would be particularly useful. In the past she had a high incidence of Chlamydia pneumoniae confirmed by medical tests, which could stand behind auto-immune diseases, when the organism destroys its own organs, such as a malfunction in the thyroid gland, or asthma. Antibiotics cannot completely remove Chlamydia pneumoniae, which has its base from spreading in the lungs. She also had troubles with her joints – another auto-immune problem, where Chlamydia could play an important role.*

- *Why the low potency of 1.5 liters? She has "irreversible" damage to her vital inner organ, the lungs, and she is no longer young. Therefore, low vitality, low potency.*
- *Why such a short interval? A lot of things have gone worse for her lately; the dynamics of disharmony are high. The increase to 2 liters could bring a somewhat longer lasting effect; this is why the interval can be increased.*
- *Why having the follow-up interview after two months? I took into account her long-lasting disease and her relatively high age; it could take some time before she reacts.*

At the follow-up I found out that she had begun the autopathic treatment a fortnight after visiting me. She told me that the headache had immediately gone worse, but then it started to improve; now it is better than when she first came – she had gone through the *healing crisis*. She also told me that tinnitus – the humming and whistling in her ears – had gone away. She had tinnitus for five years and it had been very strong, so much so that she would hear it constantly, and even in heavy noise outside. During the initial interview last time she had not mentioned it because she knew from doctors that it is incurable, and she probably did not want to waste time on it, even though it was, in her own words, "horrible". Now she has not had it at all for a month. The asthma – all its symptoms such as breathlessness, whistling in her lungs while breathing, and coughs – has gone. She can walk several miles with her dog, which she could not do before. The tingling in her arms had improved first a lot, but the last 14 days it has gone worse again. Psychologically she felt better immediately, but together with her arms it has gone somewhat worse again. She is having a lot of dreams, very vivid ones; she wakes up in a dream in a lovely place, where she feels good, under a lot of light. So she is having what are called *lucid dreams*. I had read once, it could have been in the *Washington Post*, an article by an author who had gone through a week-long course in lucid dreaming. The course was costly, and only one of the participants had managed to have a lucid dream during it. This lady had achieved it spontaneously; however she certainly was helped by meditational practice, when she used the yoga nidra in times of insomnia, which is a calming meditational technique on the boundary between sleeping and the state of wakefulness. Autopathy had cleared the way for her, in the direction she wants to take.

She did not even mention the problems with sleeping, so strong before, which usually means that the person sleeps well. Even before the first visit she suffered from an itchy back, which has become stronger together with removal of the asthma symptoms. There has even, against the cured bronchial tube, appeared redness in her skin, which she has never had before. What we are witnessing here is the working of Hering's Laws. Inside, the vitally important organ – the lungs – improved, while on the outside, the skin, in its vicinity, there is a temporary worsening. The pathology, disharmony, is being chased from the inner organ outside, from *within outward*. She once had some problems with her gall bladder, now there was a slight echo of this – the return of an old symptom. A temporary slight reappearance of an old symptom always means that the person has gone onto the path leading away from the pathology. It shows that there is a holistic tuning-up to the previous states that were once there in health, before the treatment. These symptoms never last long, most often they come in the form of a detoxification display (rash, sometimes discharge, light pain), and while the tuning-up continues, they disappear. The stiffness in her neck has improved. The pain in her hips and knees is the same as at the beginning. The heartburn has gone. The tingling in the heart area ceased immediately, but recently came back twice.

The changes came unusually fast; they are deep and very intense. The life force is strong here; despite of not appearing so at *the beginning: there is a fast succession of tuning-up. Asthma disappears in 14 days, something that with other, even younger, people had lasted six months or longer. By the first follow-up examination, removed are tinnitus, together with asthma thought to be incurable, and which even in homeopathy (let alone ordinary medicine) is a tough proposition. The area of lucid dreaming was opened, which is highly regarded in many spiritual traditions. Other things have settled down, but some of the previously improved symptoms have begun to get somewhat worse in the last 14 days. This means that **the strength of the 2 liter potency is weakening, and the amount of water needs to be increased**, to maintain the curing effect. At the same time it is possible to somewhat increase the interval of application.*

Recommendation: Continue with 3 liters every fifth day, or more often, depending on your own feeling.

I have not seen the lady any more, but as she told me, she had read my previous two books about autopathic self-treatment. I hope that she continues to expand her remarkable self-healing abilities, and has not stopped after the cure of asthma, tinnitus, insomnia, and heartburn.

The case of a skeptic, BB

Middle aged man, a technician. At the beginning of the interview, for the sake of fairness, he says to me that autopathy does not suit him philosophically, but that his wife went through the course and he let himself be talked into seeing me as a consultant. He has resolved to try it, even though he "doesn't believe in it much".

Once a month his ear canal gets blocked, sometimes the right, at other times the left and he has problems hearing. The ear canals are unpleasantly itchy every day. He has had an infection several times. It is triggered by washing, and particularly by bathing. He is allergic and sensitive to pollen; from the end of March until May his eyes get swollen, he has hay fever, and breathing problems. He is allergic to the sun, and after even slight sunburn he gets rashes on his neck and hands. He is also allergic to some foods, his throat burns and he has problems with breathing after eating an apple, banana or a peach. This is something he has had since childhood. Once a week he gets a headache from the morning and a painkiller usually fixes that. Sometimes he has stomach pains from stress.

The history: Twice he has had pneumonia – two years ago and ten years ago. He has a blocked throat twice a year, for about a fortnight. In winter he has dry eczema on the back of his hand – something he had even a week ago.

Recommendation: BB once every 14 days, first 6 liters, the next 9 liters, and after those 12 liters.

- *Why breath with boiling? Allergies are one of the many problems where the origin of the disease is not really well known. Why does the immune system in one person fight with the innocent pollen that has always been here, while with the next person nothing like this happens? Allergy is a relatively new chronic (incurable) disease, which is spreading rapidly and affects a large and growing part of population. With diseases of unknown origin, or when we suspect an auto-immune origin (organism attacks its own organs), we always choose BB as the first method of preparation.*

- *Why starting with 6 liters? The man has no problems with his inner organs; he has been having medical examinations from time to time, so his condition is therefore confirmed. The problems are only of a superficial nature. He gives the impression of robustness, and success in his profession points to his high vitality.*
- *Why the interval of 14 days? The problems have been here for many years, the worsening of the condition is only very slow. Therefore the longer interval. Why increase to 9 and 12 liters? I sometimes choose these gradual increases by 3 liters exactly in people with high vitality, when no structural changes have been found in the physical organism – when there is "only" some disruption to the functions.*

Follow-up interview in a month and a half: There was no longer any stomach pain, the itching in his ears improved, and no changes to the other problems. The preparation he probably made in longer intervals, as thus far he only took 6 and then 9 liters BB. **Continue once in three weeks 12 liters, then 15 liters BB.**

Follow-up interview in a month, end of April, in the third part of his pollen season. The allergies are substantially lesser than they used to be, except for a short episode when he was swimming in a pool. That was when his ears had briefly worsened, itching, while he had also a head cold.

The stomach was without problems. The headache was unchanged, it hurts once a week. **Recommendation: BB, 16.5 liters, repeat in 14 days.**

Follow-up in another two months. He took the recommended AP only once a month. The last one he had a couple of days ago. This year's pollen season was the best he remembers; in contrast to other years he had no breathing problems. He did not mention his food allergy, so presumably there was none. He is not complaining about a headache either. The ears are fine; recently he had a swim in the pool, and nothing – very unusual.

Recommendation: Wait and watch, 16.5 liters BB only if any previously cured problems return. On parting he told me that during ordinary work meetings, he recommends autopathy to people whom he does not even know too well. He accepts that it is a useful thing.

Self-treatment – choosing the best way of making a preparation according to feelings, SB

An obviously overweight lady comes to the first consultation with a forthcoming and supportive expression. She has already had experience with autopathy. She attended my course two months ago, and had begun to use it even after the first sitting. For thirty years she has been suffering from strong diarrhea, with light runny stool, sometimes she has to go to the toilet five minutes after a meal. Cream makes it worse, and contrary to this, meat is good for her – she likes smoked meat products. From her twenties (and she is over fifty now) she has suffered from repetitive migraines. Before autopathy she also had strong depression. She began her self-treatment with **saliva boiled, 3 liters**, she applied the preparation twice a week, and the depression had gone away after the first application. Soon she had felt much better – the chronic joint pains had improved remarkably, and she says that her psyche is 100% better. "I feel great; I'm above matters and at ease," she says. She has had no migraines since beginning to use autopathy; before that they came frequently and from the early morning. "I had suffered from heavy chronic fatigue; that has improved by 50%." She had seen improvement in her gall bladder, which used to be quite painful sometimes. The diarrheal stool, though somewhat improved, persists. Rashes in her face are improved. She said to me that soon after beginning with her self-treatment, she had once made the boiled breath – but had felt worse, so she went back to the boiled saliva, which she has been taking up till now twice a week, still with 3 liters. Even though she is very happy with what has happened in a mere two months, she would like to consult with me about what to do next. I told her to continue the self-treatment as before: the three parameters (*potency, method of preparation, and period of application*) were selected marvelously, as they have been moving the case forward. I made her aware of the possibility that this set-up might get tired – the improvements could cease, and it would be necessary to increase to 4.5 liters, with the same method of preparation with boiled saliva, which she had at the beginning compared with boiled breath, and thus found out which is better for her.

Movies in head, P2

A lady, well over eighty years old. At the first glance she looks very lively. She is exceptionally healthy, active, and she looks after her garden. She often thinks of her dear ones; she worries about them. She is also fearful when walking in the street, and at other times: fear is her constant companion. It was not like this always. She imagines some negative events that might befall those near her all the time. "I have movies in my head that I can't stop," she says. She sleeps badly; at night such thoughts are more bothersome than during the day. She also suffers from bloating, but it is not about the physical problems, which she probably has, that she wants to talk about. She wants to resolve the state of her mind.

Recommendation: Prana 2 (after dilution drop onto the forehead, then hold back in the seventh chakra, then hold also in the sixth chakra), 1.5 liters, once a week.

Follow-up interview in six weeks: The movies, the whirlpool of negative thoughts, disappeared after the first application, and thus far have not come back. She goes to sleep faster and sleeps better. Her fear has considerably subsided. She is as active as before. She says that her sore finger on her hand stopped hurting her.

She has resolved her problem – and did not come any more. The recommendation at the end of follow-up was: Prana 2, 2 liters, once a week. Sometime afterwards she sent me a letter, stating that the goal was achieved and further consultations are not needed.

How many people these days have, in various degrees, such horror movies in their heads? Perhaps all of us, with some exceptions. It can be switched off.

The case of sobbing lady, P5

A middle-aged lady came to me. It was very difficult to communicate with her and find out what was actually wrong with her. After the first few words, she began to weep, sob and sniffle, so it was almost impossible to understand what she was saying. People do sometimes cry during the interview, when they talk about their misfortunes and diseases. It is not that unusual. I therefore went for a pair of time-proven resources: I pushed a box of tissues her way, and gave her a glass of water, which sometime helps. Not in this case, however. The tissues were disappearing, so did the water, but not the tears. At the same time, I found this strange. As far as I could understand, she was not talking about any life tragedies. She had no ghastly physical illness. She had a good education and profession, her life was centered on her two small children… She told me her life story – there was nothing sinister about that either. On the contrary, someone else could easily tell a similar life story with humor and even a touch of pride. She talked about things that someone else could tell with a smile on their face. However, important was not what she said, but how she was feeling. Independent of what was going on around her, she felt immense sadness. A psychologist would probably call it depression. In such situations I have sometimes thought about what causes depression and why so many people are afflicted by it. There are various materialistic-chemical theories, but the one I hold – what else – is idealistically-pranic. Such a feeling of deep inner misfortune appears when we feel that our out-of-tune system of body and mind ceases to be able to correctly accept prana, the life force. It begins to lose contact with the higher organizational fine-matter sphere. Out of this comes anxiety and premonition of health disasters. Indeed, with further disharmony these could come, and for exactly the same reason – the cause is being out-of-tune with reception of vital information. I gave her the printed article **Prana – a simple method of self-treatment** (page 74). She was to begin with **Prana 5** (descending and ascending contactless application to all chakras), 1.5 liters. I requested that she keep records.

A follow-up interview was held in six weeks. I saw a self-confident and smiling lady, of whom I was convinced that I had never seen before, and therefore treated her as a new client. She surprised me, however, when she confirmed that she had seen me and not that long ago, and that she was "the one who constantly cried". She gave the impression of being a different person. Straightaway at the beginning, her mood was better and feelings of being unhappy about herself had disappeared. She relaxed and there came a sense of harmony. The improvements after the 1.5 liter treatment had lasted only three days, after that the bad thoughts returned, so she increased the potency. She had begun to go to a well, where she would hold the AB under the stream for 60 seconds. In that time, 2 liters of water go through the bottle. She found out that after this degree of dilution the good feelings and lack of negative thoughts lasted for a week, until the next application. With P5, immediately after making preparation and applying it, she felt some stomach pains, which had disappeared after a time and did not come back. Once she had also felt the kidneys, which was a problem that she had encountered before in life (an old symptom). Even before autopathy she had measured the pH of her urine with litmus paper, and it turned out to be very acidic. Now it is always around seven, on the boundary between acidic and alkaline, therefore the acido-basic balance has settled down even without a change of diet. She did not have the feeling of being thirsty (she was previously dehydrated). Now she spontaneously drank more, and gone were the constant thoughts about food and hunger! She is very happy, she calls it a radical change, and it has much improved her self-confidence. One could tell that at one glance. Recommendation: **Continue with Prana – a simple method of self-treatment, and increase the potency only when the previous one begins to lose effect.**
Follow-up interview two and a half months after the previous one. After about two months of good development, she had

begun to have some fluctuations – the headaches returned sometimes, and for a day, after some conflict, also the depression. She changed the bottle for a new one, and continued with the same potency, 2 liters (60 seconds of flow). The headache disappeared and so did the depression. This proved that *the bottle needed to be changed after only two months, rather than the recommended average of three.* The reason is simple; between the state of her health before the first application and after two and a half months of application, there was a big difference. From this and similar cases we deduce that **after a radical change in condition it is desirable to change bottle for a new one, because the glass retains the information about the previous states, including the one before treatment begins**. In time an old bottle reduces the effectiveness, or vibrational similarity, of the preparation. She had also tried to increase the time of flow to 120 seconds, but after that she felt tensed and irritated, had bad dreams with wild chases by terrorists. She returned to 60 seconds and all was fine again. She feels good by the spring, where she makes the preparation. Recommendation: **Increase, up to 120 seconds of flow (4 liters)**, as it is likely that she would now be better prepared for the above mentioned potency follow the previous ones, which was not the case when the first attempt to increase was made.

Follow-up a further two and a half months later: She took **120 seconds of flow (4 liters)** every one-to-two weeks, and she felt good all this time. There was no migraine, no depression, no clogged throat, from which she also used to suffer. The constant sense of being hungry, which she had before autopathy, is gone. Attention: **Hope for people who are overweight** (which she is not). My advice: Continue in this way, always bearing in mind **Prana – a simple method of self-treatment**.

The case of the laughing lady, or ten years of autopathic self-treatment

A lady, over fifty years of age – but looking about fifteen years younger – told me about her self-treatment, which had begun in 1996, after attending my lecture about holistic homeopathy. Immediately after I published my first book on autopathy in 2004, she had begun to use this brand new method. In the video called *Ten Years of Autopathic Self-treatment*, in the Testimonies section at www.autopathy.com, she says that she originally used preparations of saliva, then breath, after that saliva with boiling, then breath with boiling, and subsequently autopathy from prana. She describes how, when she had made the preparation from prana the first time. "I had this amazingly marvelous sense of lightness before going to sleep, and from the morning till noon I was laughing," she says. From morning till lunchtime she walked around the school where she teaches, and her colleagues were asking her what had happened to her to make her laugh at everything, the children were also commenting on her constant laughing. "And I couldn't stop, I just kept smiling at everything and it was very pleasant." About a month later, this time in the garden, she again made autopathic preparation using Prana 5. She adds: "When applying it I felt great warmth on all the chakras, like someone using an oxyacetylene torch on you, so strong was this feeling. It was pleasant, and also surprising, how much could happen when I only have a bottle with water with me, and nothing's happening but I still feel the unbelievable warmth." She has always had this feeling in the chakra next to which she held the bottle, and also while moving both down and up through chakras. After that, nothing out of ordinary happened and she "just" had the sense of wellbeing. How did her autopathy go over those ten years?

"I always had a good sense of wellbeing after autopathy, the boiled breath helped me much, I kept feeling good energy-wise, and with no significant slumps health-wise." Even that visit in my consultancy office was only a single one. In fact, she came to tell me that she is healthy, and that she needs no advice from me. She continues with the self-treatment, or rather in *self-harmonization*, and one can tell that she is harmonic. By the way, she is a musician. Each year I meet her a few times at various autopathic seminars, and she always assures me that she is fine. A beautiful example of how autopathy can become a part of a lifestyle, and what it can do for a person.

A chronic liver disease, eight years on autopathy, B and BB

A slim blond woman, over fifty years of age. She had an auto-immune liver disease diagnosed two years ago. Regular tests on her liver look very bad, for instance the GMT level is thirty times larger than the upper level of normality. Other values of laboratory tests also show large damage to her liver – ALP, ASP, ALT, LDL, HDL, bilirubin, all significantly above the norm. She takes medication, which she was told cannot cure the disease or even notably improve it, and that the only chance is a liver transplant. Her blood sugar levels are over, at 7–10 mmol. She suffers from strong itching felt under the skin; it is supposed to be associated with liver disease. She has scleroderma. "Lifelong" repetitive migraines. She suffers from insomnia, wakes up often, sometimes falls into sleep only after several hours of wakefulness. She is interested in esoteric matters, lives a quiet life. Since childhood she has been having a repetitive dream in which she is wandering through an old empty dark factory and cannot find an exit. We will see if she could find that exit door after all.

Recommendation: Breath without boiling, 1 liter, once a week.
I probably would have recommended BB, if that technique had been known at the time. Nevertheless, we can see that even without boiling it went excellently from the beginning. We could even speculate that if there was no boiling the case would have still developed well, but these are "maybes" that really do not belong here.

Follow-up interview in a month's time. She feels good. Even the first day after the application her small joints were sore, and she felt more tired, but that was gone the next day. After the second application in a week, the itching under the skin intensified, it was strong, the next day it passed away and had not come back. **Continue in the same way.**

Three weeks after that she had back pains and she was again tired, recommended to **increase AP from breath to 2 liters once a week**.

Two months later I learn that she had tests and that her liver levels had surprisingly improved. For instance, the GMT value had dropped to one third of the bad value she had before. Other values had also moved closer to norm, and bilirubin fell to the normal level. She has been taking the same medication for two years and nothing like this had happened. She thinks that she can see better, she can knit without glasses, which previously she could not. Sometimes her back hurts. The insomnia is gone altogether. She has not felt the itching under the skin for a long time. **Continue B, 2 liters, once weekly**.

After three months we routinely increased to **3 liters B**, and she was doing fine. She was taking this till the next follow-up, which came approximately a year after her first visit. Further tests on her liver showed the levels moving towards the norm. For instance, GMT dropped to a fifth of the original high value. The doctors ceased to talk about liver transplantation, and are showing surprise over the unexpected development. There is no insomnia. No tiredness. She used to be allergic to dust. Now she cleaned the attic and did not even sneeze. The sugar level is now around seven, before it was up to ten, but she is on no diet. **Continue 3 liters B once a week**.

Here I want to remind that if a case shows an overall movement to the better, we do not change the setting-up of our three parameters.

Follow-up in two months: GMT is worse, but still at one third of the original level. Bilirubin however is further improved. She has a lot of energy – she had unloaded and processed a load of firewood. She says she feels like being thirty years old again. *Nevertheless, even though she feels great, we can see a slight aggravation of the important liver value. Therefore, the time has come to think about changing one of our three parameters, namely the way of making.* Recommended: **boiled breath (BB), 3 liters, once a week**.

Follow-up in five months. She feels good. "Sleep is groovy," she states, and her skin does not itch. There were no migraines, nor had she had her allergies, and the splitting of her nails stopped, which was supposed to have been a sign of liver damage. She surprised the optometrist, because without glasses she could read even the next to last line, while two years ago she could not manage even the fourth last. Recommended: **BB, 3 liters, once a week.**

I will only describe further development of several years briefly. On average there were two follow-ups a year. The liver tests have held on to the improved values, some blood levels have moved to normal. The doctor told her: "There is a 95% certainty that you would not need a new liver." Usually, according to him, with her initial state a transplant is essential within a year. She stayed on BB, but the potency was slowly increased to **nine minutes under the filter (18 liters) once every 14 days.** Her sense of wellbeing was constantly being improved; she repeatedly stated that she felt great, even though there was some fluctuation in the values of her liver tests. The quality of her sleep was excellent, and the itching under the skin – so annoying before autopathy, she no longer felt. The skin on her hands had improved, which used to be scaly (before autopathy this was diagnosed as scleroderma), now it is no problem.

It is possible that this case has reached the state when move to a higher potency breath without boiling would be possible (for instance 20 – 30 liters) and the system "wait and watch", or more likely to repetitive application in longer periods, for instance once a month.

A lady and her boss, BB, P5

A woman, about fifty. She is a gentle lady, suffering from anxiety or even depression, with very low self-esteem. She had eczema and an evil boss. He would come to her from time to time, to vent his anger at her, particularly when something went wrong in the business. Such outpourings apparently calmed him down, or maybe it improved the damage to his self esteem, but at the expense of our lady – in other words, a parasitic relationship. She had always gotten worse after that, suffering from anxiety, palpitations of heart, and it took her many hours to recover.

She was taking autopathy **BB, first 3 liters, then gradually up to 7.5 liters and then alternatively with Prana 5** *(according to Prana – a simple method of self-treatment, beginning at 1.5 liters)*, once a week. The scenes her boss made soon ceased to bother her, the anxiety had gone and her role of a victim was no longer there. Consequently, his raging outbursts at her had slackened – he was forced to find himself another victim.

Whenever we use autopathy and begin to manage our case, the world becomes a friendlier place – the world in fact to a large degree mirrors the state of our mind. While we cannot directly change the world, we can change the state of our mind. Also, the state of our body – her eczema was cured shortly after commencement of autopathy.

Cancer, allergy, high blood pressure, sore knee BB, SBB, P5

A man, whom doctors had diagnosed with cancer of the lymphatic nodes. He started on **1.5 liters, BB, daily**. He soon stopped coughing, after a few days his knee ceased to hurt, which was bound for a total endoprosthesis, and he no longer felt pain in area under his right ribs. After that he came out with a normal blood pressure, though it used to be high for a long time. He no longer felt tired and his legs did not feel "like they were made of lead". After 12 days of applying AP he said that he felt better, but ever since he was told the diagnosis by his doctor, he has to urinate every half hour during the day and every hour at night-time, which he finds very annoying. He has also lost 7kg/15.4lbs of weight. It was therefore appropriate for him to eat sufficiently and give priority to alkaline foods, such as vegetables,[1] and not to allow any further slimming. Loss of weight would be threatening to him. He began to take a small spoonful of sodium bicarbonate[2] on an empty stomach twice a day in the morning and evening, dissolved in tepid water together with a spoonful of black molasses, allowing an hour before eating. Thus far he had not undertaken any conventional therapy. He ate a lot of vegetables and avoided sugar (except molasses with soda). **BB to be increased by one bottle every week (by 1.5 liters) till he gets to 6 liters.**

A month later: Thus far he used to take BB **1.5** and later 3 liters. The urinating is still very frequent, almost the same as before. Since beginning autopathy, he needs less sleep; previously he slept a lot, also during afternoons; since the first day

---

[1]   According to some experts, for instance Nobel Prize laureate Prof. Otto Wartburg, cancer is largely supported by chronic sourness of the organism and its low pH. There are number of books available in bookstores on dieting and lifestyle about how to keep pH high, alcalic.

[2]   An alkaline food supplement, baking soda, used also as food, neutralizes the acids not only in stomach, but indirectly elsewhere in body. It is a compound that our body itself creates, but not always in a sufficient quantity.

of taking AP he needs less sleep. Today he had radiotherapy for the first time.

Recommendation: Every morning saliva and breath with boiling (SBB) 3 liters, Prana 5 in the evening. P5 to begin with 1.5 liters, repeat if there is a positive change in feelings, if there is not, increase by 1.5 liters each time and wait for three days before evaluating own feelings, not to exceed 6 liters (see Prana – a simple method of self-treatment, page 74).

Follow-up examination in five weeks. The radiation therapy of his tumors was completed four days ago. He still urinates often, up to eight times a night. After the first application of P5 he was cheerful, after that he felt no change, but continued with 1.5 liters without increasing dilution. He took SBB as recommended, both daily. In six weeks he is to go to a CT scan and further examination; he has no other conventional therapy now. Recommended: once a day alternating one of these: **Prana 5, increase to 3 liters and BB 4.5 liters, and after a week increase Prana to 4.5 liters, after 14 days increase to 6 liters and at the same time increase BB to 6 liters; after 14 days increase both by 0.5 liters, and in 14 days go to 9 liters both BB and P5, still once a day, keep alternating.**

Follow-up in a month and a half. "Everything has improved," he says. Physically he feels good. He is to go to the doctor's tests only in a month's time. He does not think of the disease at all. He could "give away" energy, he says. The urinating has improved significantly, during the night he goes three times, during daytime it is now normal. The blood pressure is 130/80, within the norm. He used to suffer in spring from strong allergy; but this time it came only for two days and then left altogether. He does autopathy every day and alternates **6 liters BB and 6 liters Prana 5**, he changed three weeks ago from 4.5 to 6 liters. Recommendation: **Continue with the same values, but in case of a decline in psychology, increase both to 7.5 liters.**

Follow-up in a month and a half. He was told the results of the medical tests. Everything is in order; there was no pathological find on the CT, in blood or elsewhere. He alternates 6 liters P5 and BB, one day this, the other day that. There was no allergy, except for two days – for the first time in many years, which could hardly be the doing of radiotherapy, the same for the improved blood pressure and soreness in his knee. He is no longer chronically fatigued. He used to have to urinate within 10 minutes after he felt the need. This is no longer so, and the urinating has the normal frequency during the day, and twice during night. He had gained 2kg/4.4lbs. **Apply AP every second day and alternate 6 liters P5 and BB.**

We have communicated a few more times. He felt good, with no frequent urination, he worked full time and travelled. About six months later I recommended **increasing from 7.5 to 9 liters, with leaving three days between alternative applications, meaning every fourth day either Prana 5 or BB.**

A few months later he cancelled a scheduled visit over the phone, stating that he is very busy with work and that there was now no need for consultation. Was it a treatment of cancer? No. It was a treatment of life force.

Good karma, BB, SBB, P5

The following case illustrates what I call karma (see also Questions and Answers, page 207). Into the consultation came an enfeebled and very thin lady on crutches and with retinue. She was then eighty-seven years old. She said that she had recently spent four months in hospital, after having broken her leg at the knee. In hospital she was not drinking or eating; she had infusions, and while there she had stopped moving. Now she is beginning to eat and she is moving a bit. She has an enlarged spleen and two cysts on her uterus. The smaller cyst is to be operated on in about a month, the larger one is beyond the doctors' abilities. For twenty-seven years she has had a serious fault in blood creation called *polycythemia vera*. The doctors presume that the incurable blood disease is of genetic origin, and it can cause a multitude of other physical problems, including a cerebrovascular mishap she has suffered seven years ago. She has a disease of her thyroid gland. She cannot hear well in her left ear. She is taking a lot of medication and artificial hormones. She used to be a workaholic; now she cannot do anything.

Recommendation: BB, 1 liter, once a week.

Breath with boiling is the basic method of preparation when "the immune system" destroys its own organs, or when from the view of conventional medicine there is no known "cause" of a chronic disease, or a "genetic" origin is suspected. (The basic cause from our point of view, however, is always and in every case being an out-of-tune state towards the reception of life-force, or prana.) These days the word "genetic" is often being used as a more modern substitution to the word chronic, both of which from a practical point of view can be translated as "incurable". 1 liter was recommended because here the pathology reaches very deep into the organism, of somebody with low vitality and advanced age. The interval of one week is here because through treating many people over eighty, I found out that the low potency over a longer period usually works well here. The interval of one week is quite reliable, and applying an AP more often is not necessary. Nevertheless, with the continuing treatment we usually increase the potency, though not by more than 1.5 liters.

There was a follow-up interview held after seven weeks. She said that she feels "great, it's an enormous leap". Then she thought a little, even cried a little, and then said: "I felt a great relief immediately after application, a relief and joy… as God's blessing…" Then she quickly composed herself and continued, matter-of-factly: the tiredness had gone. Even on the second day after application, the block that prevented her from walking disappeared, and the pain in the knee that had held her mainly in bed for the past six months had gone away "as if some ring that clutched her had cracked". She stopped using crutches at home. She could breathe better and she felt a desire to be working again. Then the hearing in her left ear had gone worse, which she has had since the stroke she had years ago. But in a few days it had improved and was then better than before autopathy (we call such an aggravation prior to a significant improvement "the healing crisis")! Anorexia is gone. She has a lot more verve for housework. She went through a pre-surgical examination about a month ago, it was for a laparoscopy of a cyst planned before autopathy commenced. After this examination, a small panic broke out in the hospital – the doctors were sending her documentation back and forth, obviously suspecting that there was some confusion. It turned out that her incurable, twenty-seven yearlong diagnosis of a faulty blood cell creation may no longer be valid. The blood tests, for the first time in twenty-seven years, were normal! Then the surgery came and she had, after a single day, recovered and continued applying AP once a week. Recommendation: **BB, 1 liter, once a week.**

In our experience, elderly people usually react to autopathy more slowly, the treatment lasts longer, and we do not expect fast changes. But there was an enormous change to her psyche even after the first application, a great relief, "as God's blessing". People oftentimes say that when they first used autopathy they felt euphoria, great relaxation, or lightness. But not all of them. And also, to those that do, this pleasant phenomenon came only once at the beginning, not at all, or seldom. It is caused by a sudden change in feelings, by establishing contact with the higher fine sphere, the life force. We get used to it later, and after further applications this sudden effect usually (bar some exceptions) does not come. In this case we see everything being cured in accordance to Hering's Laws: First of all the psyche, relaxation and departure of anxiety, hopelessness, fear, then what had restricted her socially and psychologically – the inability to walk. Only after this the hearing problem was being solved, preceded by a short healing crisis. And even a month after commencing autopathy, the cells of her bone marrow had been cured – gone was the fault in blood cell creation, an unprecedented phenomenon. I am asking myself, why is it so that this very seriously ill lady, at an age close to ninety, moves so quickly towards bigger harmony, and this even on the physical level. Why is she showing almost immediate signs of improvements that go this far?

The answer: Because she has an exceptionally good karma, the readiness of the inner fine-matter system to make connection with its life force, the higher organizational principle, upon immediately receiving information on how to do it, when the resonance occurs. The good karma in this sense is a kind of "pre-harmonization", a good condition of the fine inner sphere, even though the physical one might be, for instance due to old age, decrepit. Recommendation: **BB, 1.5 liters, once a week.**

Follow-up interview in a further two months. A month ago there was a surprising improvement in the sight of her right eye. This was exactly confirmed by an optometrist. She can see well. She went again to the control testing to the hematologist: The blood tests are, for the second time, normal; the incurable disease of blood cell creation is, after nearly thirty years, not there anymore. There was stabbing pain in the knee, but that had passed in three days (old symptom reappearing). She walks at home without crutches. Her mood is good and she is not tired. Recommendation: **BB, 2 liters, once a week**. *All the improvements from the last follow-up examination have held, and some more were added. The prudent increasing of water by half a liter had proved successful, so I continue with it.*

Follow-up interview four months after the previous one. Soon after the previous follow-up her digestive system had gone worse for 14 days – it reminded her of her stay in hospital just before autopathy, but that was much stronger then, and had lasted for four months. When the short episode passed, she had again been experiencing euphoria after each application of AP. About two months ago she increased the amount of water to **2.5 liters**. After each application she felt more energy and revived. After that came a productive cough, for which she got antibiotics, and it passed relatively quickly. The repeated blood tests were still good. A month ago she increased the potency to **3 liters of water, BB**. Then I recommended her to change the way of preparation, because of the (although past) digestive problem. *Saliva can be closer to it than breath*: saliva, breath, boiling, **SBB, 3 liters, once a week**.

For a while the digestive problems appeared, as something that can be described as an old symptom reappearing – a former state that becomes evident and again disappears in the direction of cure "from within outward" (Hering's laws, page 50). It proves (which the symptoms in reverse order generally do) that the case is holistically developing to higher levels of health.

Follow-up in another two months: She was again at the hematologist and quotes the words of the surprised doctor: "I can't understand it, your blood picture is normal!" The feelings of increased energy were emerging, "freshness without tiredness", and her hearing has further improved. She goes out with a stick, which she now has "more for surety", she does not need it at home, and the crutches were forgotten about. We moved onto **4 liters, BB, once a week**.

In almost three years there were many examinations, so I will shorten the description now. In the following year she used to go shopping with the stick "just for surety", later she went out without a stick altogether – the way that she came to the follow-ups. The blood tests had fluctuated a little, but had returned to normal levels; all the improvements from previous follow-ups continued or deepened. She was taking BB **3 liters** and later **4 liters,** once a week. She was mostly in "a splendid mood", and said that once after the application she felt as if it "cleaned her head", without further specifying. She also had a brilliant reflection: "It improves things, but doesn't do it the way you'd like it. It does it its own way." On another occasion she said she had: "A feeling of joy and lightness, as if I was reaching towards the Universe." In spring there was, and went away, a bronchial infection, which she has had many times in life. At the yearly follow-up she feels great, not being tired, with the feeling of a "balloon filled up with energy". Recommended she takes **BB, 4.5 liters, once a week.**

At the next follow-up interview I'm told that she feels great and her breathing is "like in the mountains" (she lives in the city). But one day her large dog fell ill; she tried to lift him and her back started to hurt strongly. Gradually this had improved after applying the preparation, but the pain was persistent and improved significantly only after a few weeks. She said it is much better and she again has feelings of joy. The back pain was still appearing, but in a lesser way. She again went to the hematologist and said, "The lady doctor was happy with the normal blood count". When the pain in her spine came back (still the consequence of lifting the dog), she increased to 6 liters, it did not help, so she went back to 4.5 liters. She kept taking medication for the blood as for the previous twenty-seven years, as the doctor was reluctant to cut it off, "when her disease has been so nicely cured". She still walks without a stick, and sometimes after taking an AP she has a "sharpening of the brain", and other times "dusk passes to daybreak". I had recommended **BB, 4 liters, once a week, and in the middle of the week add Prana 5** (in another bottle, not affected by physical information), **first 1 liter, after some time increase to 2 liters.**

Why did I add Prana 5? It was to support her connection with the higher organizational level, which is to do with the workings of the seventh chakra. With demanding cases this works, it also adds energy, vitality and sometimes even joy. **The seventh chakra passes down to the physical level the picture of the whole healthy person that remains in existence on the fine level.** *Naturally, I cannot drop the BB, because of the physical pathology, where it was very effective.*

She had BB once a week. Altogether she only did Prana 5 three times; it is difficult for her to hold the bottle above her head for two minutes. She is laughing at the next follow-up, being much happier than the previous time; she walked in without a stick. The spine in her lower back hurts occasionally since the accident while lifting the dog, but it has improved a great deal. The blood is still in order. The parameters of thyroid gland have improved, according to tests. She is still on a lot of medication, but her doctor reduced the one for her thyroid gland. She laughs upon remembering how she first came to me: "I was just about ready to be put into the coffin". **BB, 3 liters, once a week.**

Thus far, the last time she had dropped in before going to a summer stay in the cottage. Up till yesterday she walked well, with the stick just for surety, but yesterday she slipped and pulled the ligaments in her foot, so she limps. **3 liters, BB, once a week or more often, in accordance to how she feels.**

During many of our talks I had recorded her with her consent for publication, and I sometimes show those recordings for instructions at teaching courses. The female students particularly love this video, and upon seeing it some even cry with joy.

Wait and watch – high blood pressure, SB

A woman with high blood pressure, and the disease began six years ago, when she had 180/120. Now she takes two kinds of pills, however, the pressure over a long time is still high above the norm. Her overall state of health has lately been sharply deteriorating, which worries her. For the last three weeks she has felt awfully tired, and the last week the veins in both legs began to "terribly" hurt, she says. She also gets strange pressure marks on her legs, which stay for two days, for instance from sitting on a park bench. These marks first appeared two months ago. In the last six months, twice a month she gets a strong headache, which she had not suffered from before. I recommended **one-off application, 6 liters, SB** (saliva boiled).

Why 6 liters? The lady sees doctors and no problems with inner organs were found. Overall she gives the impression of being dynamic and occupied. Why one-off? Because at the time I prescribed even the saliva boiled once-off, and successfully so. The beginnings of autopathy were indeed with one-off application, which I was used to from the homeopathic, so-called "Kentian" practice, which I had practiced for twenty years before autopathy, and studied and eventually taught at my Homeopathic Academy in Prague. Later, however, it turned out that in the majority of autopathic cases regularly repeated applications work more reliably, particularly when a one-off application at the beginning of treatment worked only a little. After such experiences, for a number of years I have been recommending regularly repeating the applications of AP almost every time from the beginning. However, this case came my way years ago, and for my current practice it would be somewhat atypical. Nevertheless, at the later stages of treatment I very often move onto the wait and watch system, as the potency of AP gets higher and so does the state of health.

Follow-up in a month and a half: The third day after application the soles of her feet had begun to itch, then also the palms of her hands, only in the morning after waking up. That is a new symptom for her, which she never had before. There was a small rash as well. From my homeopathic practice I knew already that small rash and itching of skin is sometimes the first sign of the departure of an inner pathology in the way "from within outward". Much had improved already. The tiredness is gone. The pain in her veins went away immediately after the AP application. The strange pressure markings also disappeared. After many years of being high, her blood pressure also settled on 130/80, in the norm. Recommendation: **SB, 12 liters, one-off.**

Follow-up in three month: She feels good, not tired, the blood pressure has dropped down further, her doctors reduced the amount of medication, she has no problems, all has gone away. Recommendation: ***Wait and watch.*** *No autopathy, things are getting better under the influence of the previous application.*

Follow-up examination in four months: She has no problems. Feels happy. Nothing happened during that time. She never took measurements of her blood pressure even once. One of the two medications was discontinued, and she takes the other in smaller doses. Recommendation: **Wait and watch, if a health problem of any kind occurs, apply SB, 12 liters, one-off.** *The lady is now in an advantageous position – she has reached the state of complete and undisturbed health, therefore it should be easy for her to see when another application is needed – simply when something is out of the ordinary.*

A one-off application followed by meticulous observations and recording of the state in the "wait and watch" phase, is also effective with the boiled preparation. The "wait and watch" system generally is the target of any treatment, as soon as things have visibly settled down. It appears, nevertheless, that in the current environment, where toxicity is on the increase, and where many toxic influences are not even felt and recognized as such, the repeated application is the standard method of combating outside disturbances.

Eczemas

While I continually stress that autopathy is never aimed at a particular disease, because it tunes-up the whole organism (which of course contains problems we want to cure), there are illnesses everywhere around us and in us. People hopelessly combat these their entire lives, while it is very easy and in many cases even quick to get rid of them. A typical problem of this nature is **eczema**. Autopathy usually catches up with it, and we have many cases that prove it. Eczemas, even those that are lasting years, strong, defacing and very annoying, react well to the autopathic process of tuning-up. I have had many in my consultancy room. It is not just that autopathy had done a service to eczematics; they also did a lot for autopathy in return. The vanishing of eczema happens to be a very obvious and noticeable change, so the neighborhood immediately takes notice of autopathy. All the methods of preparation have worked well here, though the dominating ones are SB and SBB. It is not just the people who have come to my consultancy room, but also the attendees of my lectures and readers of my books. At breaks during courses, a queue usually forms at my table, with people seeking a short answer to their problems or those of the ones they are treating.

One of them was a lady who told me how with the lower potencies the treatment of her eczema went well. But when she increased it to 6 liters, the eczema came back on her face, where previously it was already cured. I advised her to **lower** the potency to the level where the eczema had gone from her face before. Sometime later she let me know that she did not follow my advice and was determined to continue with 6 liters. However, in the morning, before she could make the preparation, her friend walked away with one of her bottles, so she was forced to lower the amount of water. And the eczema had once again disappeared. The lady concluded that nothing in the world is just chance event, that I was right about the lowering of amount of water, and that it gave her back the peace of mind. We both think that fortuities do not exist.

Another lady, who is not my client, wrote to me recently, without giving any details, that her long-time eczema had completely disappeared after two months of regular application of low potency P5.

Many children suffer from this unpleasant and painful disease, despite taking various chemical substances in the form of pills or ointments, which cannot cure their health problems. Why? The chemical preparations work only on the physical level, but the cause of the disease is not there.

Naturally, treatment of eczema is always a holistic process, it is (as always) about tuning-up the whole to reach a state of health. This process may not necessarily be entirely simple and short, it depends (as always) on the overall state of body and mind. Eczema usually is only one on the rich palette of other complaints the person being treated is having.

Switch to one-off application and the "wait and watch" system – the case of a child's eczema, SB, B, BB

The mother of a five-year-old boy told me this during the initial consultation: Atopic eczema had appeared in the first six weeks of his life, first on the head, then on his legs, and the body. It gets better during summer, and is at its worst in spring and fall. There are alternating periods of itching and non-itching. He gets pimples that he scratches, and the scabs that then form.

He is allergic, and tests have revealed that he is allergic to birch trees and to dogs. He has recurrent inflammation of the middle ear, and once or twice a year the doctor has been piercing his ear drum since he was two years of age. This is connected with a head cold and he always gets antibiotics. There is frequent nose bleeding in the boy's history, which had lasted for several years, but a year ago it abated, even though it occasionally still happens, as it did a day before him visiting me. At year and a half of age he had tonsillitis treated with antibiotics. He takes oral medication for his birch tree allergy, which still occurs every season despite the medication. I recommended **SB, 6 liters**, once a week.

- *Why 6 liters? This is the highest potency that we use to begin treatment; it concerns persons with high vitality. The boy is vital, his inner organs have not been affected, and he is resisting descending into pathology beyond the level of skin, which is on the periphery.*
- *Why SB? This method of preparation proved itself useful with skin inflammations, which often fester, there are bacteria and yeast cells.*

Follow-up in two and a half months: The skin is fine. About a month after commencing the treatment, the eczema had gone worse for a few days. For two days in this spell he had a temperature of 39°C/102°F and a headache. During the days

112

that followed he was without a temperature or pain, but had begun to cough (departure of toxins) and then got a head cold (Hering's Law – from within outward). In the end the skin was cured and the eczema was gone. Since then he has been fine for a month. I recommended not continuing with AP applications, and switching to the "wait and watch" system. This means, even though the child is healthy, his development has to be watched, and if there are signs of symptoms returning, the AP has to be applied again, in the same potency and method of making as before.

The healing crises had appeared a month after commencing autopathy, the eczema got worse and a high temperature came, but only for two days; the child stayed in bed at the time, and was given no antibiotics. After this, the toxins were being discharged in the form of a strong cough and blowing his nose. After about a week, the cleansing process came to an end, followed by a state of health, without the chronic eczema. Recommendation: **Wait and watch.**

Follow-up interview in two and a half months: A week after the previous interview, a small eczema appeared on his leg. **Applied SB, 6 liters**. It went away immediately, but it was back in 10 days. And again it disappeared on its own. *The case was developing in line with Hering's Law "from above downward". Previously the eczema was on his head, and then on his body, it went away, and lastly appeared on his leg. The application was a bit too hasty, but why not?* ***By a "hasty" application we do not spoil anything, so long as we use the same potency and same method of preparation as before.*** *And we could sometimes even help the process of treatment, as with repetitive applications. The organism, however, took over in the end, caused skin inflammation on leg, which went away on its own, and that was that.* The nose bleeding has gone altogether. The birch trees are in flower right now, which in this season used to regularly cause an allergic display. The itching was evident only for one day, whilst it used to last over the whole season. There is no eczema.

I recommended a one-off application of **BB, 9 liters**. The "wait and watch" system continues.

Follow-up examination in three months. A month after the previous visit, eczema had appeared for a short time on his leg, it disappeared, and then appeared on the hips, but only for a short time. Since then, for two months there was none. Sometimes he scratches his leg, even though the eczema is no longer there. Four times the nose bleeding came back, about a week apart, but the last month there were no problems. The happy mother says that her son has improved on all fronts, even in his behaviour and psychologically. Recommended 12 liters breath, no boiling, one-off, only if problems came back.

After that came a light head cold; while there was no eczema, it had appeared on his hips for 10 days – a warning sign. Though it was only relatively a slight one, the symptoms this time moved **from down, upwards – against Hering's Laws.** Then an occasional nose bleed came, and itching in his nose. That meant the AP should be applied, as was recommended the last time, which the mother duly did. All the symptoms just mentioned then immediately went away, and the boy was returned to health. I advised his mother to watch even over trifling problems as they could be signals of an upcoming decline and relapse (itching in nose, head cold, etc.). In such a case the preparation in the latest setup needs to be reapplied.

Follow-up a year after the last one: Three months after the mentioned one-off application of **12 liters BB,** the eczema reappeared slightly on leg. They applied **15 liters BB** (breath with boiling) and within two days the eczema was gone. He was healthy for three months, when the return of the light eczema on leg came. They applied immediately 20 liters BB, and in four days it disappeared. Throughout the year he had no acute problems, such as he used to have, and in that time he only once had a head cold (untreated). They went to have allergological tests, which this time came up clear. When the boy comes into contact with a dog it does nothing to him, whereas he used to be allergic. When the birch trees flowered this year, he had no problems. Recommendation: **Wait and watch, if eczema would appear or any other previously removed chronic problem, apply breath without boiling, 20 liters, one-off.** *No boiling, because the detoxification cure with boiled breath had already been successfully done, and the time has come to move onto the clean preparation without boiling. The potency of 20 liters is sufficiently high for it to be effective in the long-term. The AP should be applied under the system of "wait and watch", meaning only in the case of any of the already cured problems coming back.*

The boy is still being looked after autopathically by his mother, who has learned to work independently, had read books on autopathy and had been through the course. She no longer needs my advice. Her meticulous observations and detailed notes, which she had kept all this time, had returned her boy to health. A number of years have passed since our last meeting.

Crohn's disease, alternating SB and BB

A lady over forty told me that she has Crohn's disease. It is a chronic inflammation of the small intestine, with many and various consequences. It is an incurable disease that she has had for the past seven years. She is on a lot of medication, particularly corticoids. In the last year she has been very tired, and more so in the last three months. She feels as if "she was poisoned". The disease had begun with a strong abdominal pain. Now her belly hurts to touch and when running, so she had to stop doing sports. She suffers from constipation and strong flatulence with pressure onto the thorax. While the doctors' findings do not significantly change, she feels worse and worse, and lately this has been accelerating. Recently she felt very bad, and stayed home from work for a week; she was terribly tired, shaking, feeling anxiety, with breathing difficulties. Her states of anxiety are repeating. Until the disease started, she was relatively healthy. I recommended alternating **SB and BB: 1.5 liters every second day for 14 days, then 3 liters once a week, in one AB.**

I chose SB because it was an intestinal disease, a problem with the digestive system, from which saliva comes, even though it is from the other end. BB because it was an auto-immune disease. Alternating two different preparations (as opposed to joining into one in SBB) was chosen because in my experience, and some other consultants' opinions, it works more swiftly. We will never find out how the joint preparation of SBB would have worked in this particular case, but I think that it too would have been effective.

Follow-up interview in two months. After three applications she had stomach pains and flatulence. After 14 days she felt a marked improvement in everything, but particularly the psyche, and did not feel that "terrible tiredness, as if something was pushing to the ground". She still is in a joyful euphoria; everybody says that she has changed. She recently had an enormous workload, and managed it with ease. She can now eat whatever she wants; previously some foods made her condition worse. She reduced the corticoids by one-third and is fine; beforehand when she reduced the intake there were immediate intestinal problems, but not this time. She has no flatulence, which had followed her nearly all the time. She is elated, saying that there is nothing wrong with her. Formerly, she was reluctant to go to work, now she is full of vigor. I recommended continuing with the autopathy as before, i.e. **alternate SB and BB, 3 liters, once a week.**

While the setup of three parameters (potency, period, method of preparation) continues to move the case to the better, we do not change it for as long as this influence lasts. We think about changing it only if the effect of the therapy stagnates, or if there are signs of a relapse, and the return of already cured symptoms.

Follow-up in another two months: She feels good. She can eat anything without having any intestinal problems or flatulence. Physical loads do not bother her, which used to make things worse. She went for blood tests at the hospital and no problems were found, whereas previously she had a high inflammation marker. They had reduced two of her medications, which she was taking regularly. People who know her say that she has "made a 180-degree turn". She is not tired and her psyche is much improved. Recommendation: **Continue alternating BB and SB once a week 3 liters; only if the effect slackens, increase to 4.5 liters.**

Chlamydia pneumoniae

Chlamydia pneumoniae is an intracellular parasite, which attacks various cells in the human body[3] (for instance in the lungs, nerves, blood vessel walls,[4] joints, intestines, skin, kidneys, thyroid gland, etc.). Some experts think it is an important cause of so-called auto-immune diseases.[5] It is widely spread, though in the majority of its hosts it does not have to actually cause more significant health problems. However, if the organism is weakened, there could be problems, usually incurable, and usually not considered to be associated with this parasite (for instance, those auto-immune problems). The organism then destroys its own infected cells, in futile attempts to get rid of the parasite. It is impossible to remove it simply by conventional methods – not even the strongest antibiotics regularly taken for a long time usually completely remove it – and then it returns.

---

[3] www.cpnhelp.org
[4] www.ncbi.nlm.nih.gov/pubmed/28387800 "Molecular characterisation of Chlamydia pneumoniae associated to atherosclerosis".
[5] www.ncbi.nlm.nih.gov/pubmed/19151119 "Acute Chlamydia pneumoniae infection in the pathogenesis of autoimmune diseases".

Auto-immune disease, BB

A lady over fifty, who has strong and frequent headaches, *auto-immune disease of salivary glands – the saliva is not forming. She has anemia and leukopenia, she feels tired, often has acute diseases, cough, head cold, and influenzas.* Her thyroid gland was surgically removed and she takes substituting hormones. Three years ago, her Chlamydia pneumoniae levels were found to be high. And five months ago they found an extremely high level of this parasite and gave her antibiotics. At the same time **she had begun autopathic self-treatment: 3 liters, BB, once a week.** She was tested after that, and Chlamydia pneumoniae was reduced to the previous lower level, though still above norm. She came to see me, and I recommended **4.5 liters, BB, once a week. Gradually we increased this to 9 liters.** The headaches subsided and were not so frequent; her tests for anemia and leukopenia were near the norm. Three months after her first visit she reported to me that she no longer had headaches. The Chlamydia levels have been reduced from twice the norm – to back to norm. The saliva was beginning to form.

Boiled breath (BB) was appropriate to use here, because it is the most useful preparation for people suffering from auto-immune problems of any kind. For our understanding, we can consider any long-term health problem caused by the organism destroying itself to be an "auto-immune" disorder. For instance, in the form of chronic inflammation, the body destroys one of its own organs, or cells (also in joints, arteries, glands, nerves, liver...), because it knows there is an intruder. But why is it there? The basic cause is the same with all diseases: The organism is out-of-tune with the reception of prana, and it therefore cannot get rid of the intruder through its own (vital) force. Thus: Do we have a remedy for parasites? We do not! However, we could stimulate the fine-matter life force streaming to us from the Source, and reorganize the system of body and mind. As soon as the body has completely lost its ability to accept the life force, it becomes prey to microorganisms, and they take it apart.

The transition from BB to breath without boiling, and a significant increase in potency – the case of auto-immune disease

Throughout her life she has suffered from recurrent inflammations, first of the throat, then also the joints, urinary tract and her female organs. As soon as she got rid of one thing, another had begun. As far back as she could remember, she always took some antibiotics. She also had other medication, for instance against her thyroid gland insufficiently functioning. Now she is near forty years of age, she has insomnia, painful joints, allergy, osteoporosis and chronic fatigue. Psychological problems are the worst; it got worse after the doctors told her about the results of her blood tests. She has a positive (over the norm) *rheumatic arthritis, and also Chlamydia pneumoniae and trachomatis, and above all, the antibodies to lupus erythematodes,* an incurable auto-immune disease, which when fully developed can gradually destroy inner organs and be life threatening. She is now much afraid of what might be – anxiety and fear. Recommended: **BB, 3 liters, every second day.**

At the first follow-up examination she did not feel any better than the first time. Even the second and third follow-ups were not much good. Only after gradually increasing the dilution to **7.5 liters BB once a week**, was there a sudden turn. "I don't even remember when I felt this good," she said. She added that she feels an upsurge of energy, and no longer worries as much about her problems. "I'm happy to be alive again."

It improved further after increasing to **9 liters BB**. I recommended **repeating once a week for three weeks 9 liters, BB; then increasing it to 10.5 liters once a week, and then to 12 liters BB**, once every two weeks.

Two months have passed, and at her next visit with a meaningful glance, she handed me the papers with medical report: *The recent tests have shown that all the previous threats are gone* – borelia, Chlamydia pneumoniae and trachomatis, and above all, lupus erythematodes. Including rheumatic arthritis. Despite the previous tests, all that is now within the norm. Therefore, her mood and her life perspective have improved enormously. And with it receded a number of physical problems.

Nevertheless, gynecological problems (which she has had most of her life) were still there, and she usually did not hesitate to use antibiotics. Nevertheless, after a one-off application of **breath without boiling 30 liters**, all the problems disappeared almost immediately. She was as healthy as she ever was. This lasted almost a year, before she repeated the same potency from breath, when some of the problems came back slightly, but went away again.

*The moral: This method, which supports the gradual cleansing of the organism (detoxification) by increasing potencies of boiled breath, and eventually increasing to up to three-times the amount of water from **unboiled breath and transitioning the system to "wait and watch"**, has regularly been successful, with long-term and outstanding success. Even some very complicated cases can quickly stabilize, and reach a state of health, when we increase the potency to 30 or more liters, with the change to breath without boiling. However, the detoxification phase with the lower potencies of boiled breath was essential initially, and it helped her to get rid of the great threats, mainly from the resident parasites and the existence of auto-immune problems.*

Regular application of boiled preparation with subsequent significant increase of dilution and transition to unboiled breath and the "wait and watch" system

Here is another case. A middle-aged woman came to me. She was healthy up until three years ago, when arrhythmias and repeated urinary tract inflammations had begun to bother her. After this came issues with her pancreas, bloating and bad digestion. Overall she was on the downhill slide, being under extreme pressure in her professional job, in which she invested all her energy. Now she had lost all her strength, she has eczema, arrhythmias, she is very emotional, tired, ruled by sadness, says that "she feels like being at the end of the road". She knows that it cannot go on like this. Both she and her husband would have wanted a child, but conception does not occur. We began on **boiled breath with increases from 6 to 12 liters.** In time she reports that many things have improved: her emotions, arrhythmia, and eczema disappeared. Nevertheless, she continued in her demanding profession, and after a while there were relapses, panic attacks, depression, and a return of arrhythmias. Still no conception and the age of forty just around the corner. After six months of autopathy, I therefore recommend **30 liters, B** (breath, no boiling). Soon after this she also took **32 liters, B, one-off.**

Six months later she relates that she had settled down psychologically immediately after the application, the arrhythmias had gone, and the whole that time she was fine, except for work-related stress, from which she now, unlike in the past, does quickly recover. Nevertheless, still no conception. Advice: **Increase the potency from breath to 42 liters, though only if depression came back or something else from the previously cured problems.**

She did not apply an AP, and nothing came back, but in two months' time she reports that she is three weeks pregnant, which tests confirmed. In the sixth month the arrhythmias began to return, then she made **42 liters B** and it settled down. After the birth she also asked me, if she could repeat the potency from breath, with which I had agreed; childbirth usually is a stressful matter, and **repeating of previously used potency soon after delivery is almost a rule.**

This was a case of infertility, a very much widespread complaint, which these days besieges the European western population. It is a time when women have to postpone starting a family till the age of nearly forty, when it could easily be too late. Many of our experiences point out to the fact that infertility can be solved by autopathy.

In connection to this, I recall another case of a **middle aged woman**, who had a large number of chronic health problems. She took lower potencies of BB, but after applying a **30-liter** potency from breath, it all settled down. Without having to repeat the AP, she bore then a healthy child. Shortly before the birth, mycosis had appeared, but left on its own. After the birth, she had made 30 liters, breath without boiling, as I had advised her previously. As far as the child goes, she told me at the last visit: The child is healthy, does everything early. At three weeks it held its head up, which usually happens at two months; it rolled to its side at two months, which normally comes after six months; at two and a half months it moved on the bed pushing itself by the legs. Apart from its better-than-average abilities, the forty-year-old mother's child is absolutely healthy, which was not the case with its considerably older sibling.

The children of mothers who have been under autopathic treatment, or who have begun autopathy at the beginning of pregnancy, usually are healthy and well developed. It becomes prominent when compared with an older sibling, whose mother did not have autopathy before its arrival. A certain birth assistant, who is also an autopathy consultant, told us in a discussion during a seminar, that she often witnesses this effect.

From the point of view of therapeutic techniques, transitioning to higher potencies from breath without boiling is usually appropriate at the more advanced stages of treatment. It can follow preparation made of prana or a boiled preparation, particularly with potencies of 30 liters and more. This is without regard to the character of original problems; and the person's age does not play a significant role either. We will have to say more on this in Part Six.

Finding the best potency –
the case of self-treatment, S

In 2014 a young man came to me, whom I had previously last seen five years before that. He had originally started coming to my consultancy in 2005. It was then, nine years earlier, he told me that from an early age he suffered from hay fever with a clogged nose and sneezing, which always lasted from April until the end of August. At winter time he was not healthy either, with the arrival of the cold season, the head cold would move down to his chest, and a chronic cough lasted throughout winter. He also felt a chronic tiredness the whole year. His nasopharynx was congested the whole year. At winter time he had eczemas on his leg and hands. Mycosis repeatedly appeared on his groin and legs. He had head colds and even pneumonias. Inflammation of his sinus cavity came repeatedly. He even had shingles, and inflammations of the middle ear. All this was accompanied by a long-term, though interrupted, intake of antibiotics. He went through German measles, mumps and rubella, which came soon after being vaccinated against rubella. I had originally recommended **one-off** application of an **AP made of saliva, 6 liters**.

In the middle of pollen season about two months later, he reported that the sneezing was lighter than usual, and gradually he got rid of his other problems. The regular inflammation of the nasopharynx had not arrived. The skin problems were gone, only some marks remained. He felt well, and his tiredness had disappeared immediately after the application.

In two months' time the hay fever returned with all its manifestations. But after a one-off AP from saliva, 12 liters, it had gone within a week, and so he stopped taking all the pills – even then the head cold did not come back, albeit the pollen season was still on. Eczema, which he had for fourteen years, was no longer there. The next pollen season went without him taking any pills, there were only very light shows of allergy, and in the second part of the season not even these appeared.

He said that he had a summer when he felt healthy for the first time since the age of five. Only at the end of 2006 did he once repeat an AP of **12 liters saliva**. The next year he increased it to **15 liters one-off**, because the head cold returned – and it had gone away. After this he was applying an **AP of 15 liters** from saliva always one-off, once or twice a year when the head cold came, which always quickly passed. He applied about one or two preparations a year. The last potency recommended by myself was in 2009, 16 liters from saliva one-off, after a short bout of head cold.

For the next four years he had none of the serious acute diseases that had bothered him previously. And he had nothing of a chronic nature either. Therefore he correctly assumed that he no longer needed me, and moved onto self-treatment. He reappeared again after five years. He said to me that for all that time he was applying an AP once every three to four months of **16 liters saliva**, always when the slight head cold came shortly and then went away. Therefore, for five years of his autopathic activity he was healthy. He said that he had no winter colds and that common illnesses stayed away from him. Only once did he have a problem – a cough came a year ago, he had made the AP immediately – but this time it did not work, and the cough continued. He realized that he used suspiciously cheap bottled water; obviously chlorinated, and filled with the town water (these are sometimes sold as "drinking water" or similar). As soon as he returned to unprocessed spring water again, everything was fine. He says that his health is excellent. For all this time he takes his reliable potency of 16 liters saliva, which has been time-tested. Actually, he came only to have a chat with me and to ask if I happen to have some innovation, after all these years. I did. I advised him to take **breath without boiling 16 liters**, whenever he feels he needs it and continue with self-treatment as before. If, in time, this time-proven dilution began to lose its effectiveness, he should increase it by 1.5 liters. Recently I saw him on television, where he was presented as an expert; obviously he is doing well in his profession.

Creative approach – alternating SBB with P5 and applications on chakras in front and on back

A slim lady, about forty. She says that a year and a half ago she was having depression and felt that life is not worth living. She thought that it was too much for her. She had eczema, was sad and tired, and had long-term inflammation of her urinary tract, together with pains in her stomach and lower belly. She used to have blood in her urine, and for the past five years her left kidney was hurting her. The urinary tract problems had been with her from childhood, she was repeatedly taking antibiotics, which had first improved things a little, until everything quickly was returning into the previous unendurable state. To add to this, a year and a half earlier they found changes to her cervix. Her knee was sore, left groin muscle also hurt, and she had varicose veins in both legs. She had migraines that were getting worse, also allergies, hay fever, and asthma since childhood – with breathlessness, which had improved in adulthood though. There were problems with hemorrhoids; times of feebleness when she felt like fainting, dark spells in front of her eyes, and cold sweats. She had scoliosis and for a long time had suffered from back pains.

At this stage in her life she felt that she cannot go on like this – and she went to the course in autopathy. She had completed courses 1 to 3, and right from the beginning she was making APs. She began her self-treatment with **3 liters BB**, and applied it regularly and gradually increased it, so that in a year and a half she had most recently reached **60 liters, BB**.

During that year and a half, most of her chronic problems were settled: First of all her psyche improved (curing from "within outward"), then the eczema, which had shortly worsened and then quickly disappeared. In spring she was puffed up as usual due to her long-time allergy, but after increasing potency to **40 liters, BB** it went away, and for the whole of summer and fall, when the allergies used to regularly appear, she had no significant allergic reactions. The last hint of it had gone in summer, full three months before the usual end of the season, and this after increased the AP to **60 liters, BB**.

Following her self-treatment, since her first visit she has had no migraines. Gone are the constant pains in her groin and knee; varicose veins have been improving, but when they got worse she knew that she needed another dose of autopathy, which made it go away. The need for another application is also signaled to her by tiredness, which she normally does not have, and which retreats after applications. Improved were the urinary tract problems, though they still do appear. The kidneys, however, do not hurt anymore (the direction of the problems' withdrawal "from within outward"). Her menstruation has settled down, it used to always be very painful. However, after **4.5 liters BB**, she has experienced a painless one for the first time in her life. Old symptom from her childhood reappeared – shortly her ear was hurting as it used to with an infection of the middle ear, which she twice had as a child. Another test showed the previous findings on her cervix had improved. She tried also the **preparation from Prana 5**, got to 9 liters, and felt "incredibly good" psychologically. But she returned to the preparation from breath with boiling.

My advice was: Alternate **60 liters BB with P5**, which she should start on **9 liters and increase depending on how she feels, and on its effectiveness**. P5 to be taken more often, 60 **liters of BB** only occasionally, particularly if any inflammation appeared. *I have recommended this, because both these ways of application have worked in the past.*

If you alternate prana with other technique of preparation, it is not necessary for the preparations to be of the same potency. On the contrary, it has been effective to judge the effect of prana and bodily information separately, in the period immediately after applying prana, i.e., if the interval is one week, we assess how we felt in that period. If we had a positive effect, we would repeat the same potency; if there was no discernible effect, we increase it (page 74, Prana 5 and 2, simple procedure).

Preparation from prana has the advantage that its effect on the psyche can be felt very quickly, sometimes within hours, days or even sooner, if the potency was selected well. We assess the effect of BB or SBB more on a basis of longer observation, even though the feelings in the first days after application also play their role.

Follow-up examination in six weeks: She is smiling pleasantly, looks relaxed and says, "I feel wonderful". In that time she twice applied an AP of **BB, 60 liters**, and eight times **Prana 5, while increasing from 4.5 liters** (she made it differently than I advised her, but I am not upset, the intuition of the given person is an important guide). After prana she feels a great movement in the mind, from the potency of **7.5 liters** it is a big difference, and she **"feels happy"**. She takes it once a week. *The feelings of happiness are sometimes mentioned by people who have found their correct potency while applying AP from prana. The latest potency P5 was* **17 liters**, *and after that she had a slight short headache, which she ordinarily no longer gets. The urinary tract inflammation is the only thing that troubles her sometimes, but not the kidney pains. These are problems she had since childhood, so let's remind ourselves of Hering's Law number two: "The problems are being cured in the reverse order to how they appeared". The first, the oldest ones, are cured last. Recommendation:* **Prana 5, 17 liters,** *no longer applied regularly but depending on how she feels, if the improvements are waning, and in the same way adjust the potency according to feelings, add water if there is a lesser effect. Using a different bottle, apply BB, 60 liters as before, but only if there is a suspicion that there is an inflammation somewhere.*

Next follow-up in two and a half months: She continued with **Prana 5, 17 liters** once a week and she made an improvement. She was holding the potency in the vortex chamber of the AB not only in front of the body, but also at the back, and as she moved upwards through the chakras she did it first at the back and then in front – after this she experienced a strange and pleasant sensation: "As if the back was opening, it cannot be *described*. Relaxation, an upsurge of energy and happiness, but twice, the body opens up into the space." She also made **preparations**

from the forth, and then first and second chakras, by first holding the vortex chamber with water for two minutes in the chakras involved, always in front and the back, and she made the potency and took it to the same chakra – and experienced good feelings. She applied it every three days, increasing from 1.5 to 4.5 liters, and it was because of emotions and a slight disturbance in her urinary tract. Now she has had no problems with her urinary tract for two months, and the lifelong chronic pains in her lower abdomen have disappeared.

By the way, chronic cystitis, which apparently could be the diagnosis of this lady, involving the urinary tract, nowadays presents a problem that destroys the sense of life of many women and men, who after many years of suffering from constant pains usually think that there is no help for them. A month ago she had also made **SBB, 60 liters** and felt "very good". "The health problems have left me," she says and during the interview she never stops smiling. The return of this lady to her true self thus took only a little over a year and a half, and the substantial part was due to self-treatment, after a course in autopathy.

Mollusca – a simple case, SB

A year-old boy, who has small reddish vesicles under his arms and on his head. They formed two months ago, and accrued. Recently he had a head cold and now a chronic cough. On a calf he has light eczema. Doctors told his parents that in such cases the mollusca have to be removed surgically, which could be rather painful, and also without a guarantee that the problem will not return. They already tried homeopathic symptomatic remedies, but without success. Recommendation: **Saliva boiled, 6 liters; in a week's time 9 liters, and in another week's time 12 liters saliva without boiling.** Then observe.

Follow-up in five weeks. The acute problem with cough went away immediately, the mollusca stopped increasing. But they are still there. A day after a second application he had temperature, up to 38°C/100°F, that lasted four days, and a head cold that also lasted four days. Recommended: **12 liters BB** once a week, after three applications increase the interval to 14 days. Return to boiling was obvious here; **while inflammation lasts, we boil.**

Follow-up in two months: Within five weeks the mollusca had completely disappeared. So did the little eczema. He has no problems. Continue once a month with BB **12 liters**, to prevent a relapse. After three months move onto the "wait and watch" system, with no more applications of AP.

Five years, she never was healthy, BB

A mother brings to me a five-year-old girl, who had been suffering from serious abdominal problems since birth. She has such severe constipation that sometimes her bowels do not open for up to 10 days. Her usual frequency is every third day. By contrast, occasionally she goes three times a day. It has improved slightly when they stopped giving her dairy milk products. She often complains about stomach pains. There is sometimes blood in her stools. Doctors do not know why she has these problems, and none of the chronic illnesses she has had since birth have been cured by them – including the atopic eczema that came soon after her birth, nor her numerous headaches. Recommendation: **Start with BB, 4.5 liters, once a week, after two applications increase to 6 liters, BB, once a week.** *Here boiled saliva was the first choice method of preparation primarily because of the disease of digestive system, from which saliva comes, even though it is from the other end.*

Follow-up in two months: There was blood in her stool only once since our last meeting, and at the beginning of the treatment. The constipation had gone away immediately, and since then her bowels have been opening regularly once a day. And now they can even give her food that used to make things worse, such as chocolate or ice cream. She only complained about stomach pains at the beginning of the treatment, and not anymore. In the first three weeks there were some headaches, four times altogether, but not after that. There is no eczema. Thus her mom had brought to me – even for the first follow-up – a healthy child, cured from the numerous and "incurable" diseases. Because this state of good health was here only a short while, it was necessary to **repeat the preparation at an increased interval in a dilution of 6 liters once every 14 days, to prevent a relapse.**

Follow-up examination in another four months: The mom reports that the state of good health continues, even though the last application came only after three weeks. I told her that I advise applying **BB, 9 liters, once every 14 days**, to maintain the state of good health.

Two years later the mother asked me about an acute infection that her daughter currently had. It turned out that in the meantime she was without problems, even though for most of the time she had no autopathic treatment. I recommended a return to what has worked in the past so well: **BB, start on 6 liters. Apply AP repeatedly for a time, if needed increase to 9 liters.** *Acute disease usually is the first sign of a beginning overall out-of-tune state, which without treatment could continue and cause a return of chronic problems.*

The right not to think, P5

Our civilization is burdened by a disease that brings us a lot of suffering: we think needlessly. Some of us live in a virtual world of thoughts, fantasies, desires, fears and worries, and only very few perceive the real present moment, which may not be anywhere near as bad as we imagine it.

A lady over fifty came to me for an autopathic interview. She is unhappy. She continuously thinks about a relationship that ended many years ago. She was happy in it. But after her partner's departure, she is grieving. She has to work hard trying not to think about it. She has to keep proving to everybody that she is very happy and useful. But she feels lonely. She does not know how to relax. She helps her daughter and grandchildren, they think it suits her, but she is annoyed by not having her own life. She has chest pains in the heart region, her gall bladder hurts, she is losing hair, a twitch in the eye, headaches, fungus on the nails, and cramps in her legs. She cannot drive her car, because she is scared. All is lost. She often weeps, even now as she is telling me about it. Nevertheless, doctors maintain that she is healthy! I had recommended her an AP of **Prana 2** from the seventh chakra. It connects us to the higher levels of the Universe, and this is how she should be treated.

The AP was to be repeated once a week and dilution gradually increased. She had started on 3 liters, she was to repeat each dilution twice, and then increase it by 1.5 liters.

She came again in a month. She kept laughing and told me that the sadness had largely left her, which was quite visible. She can relax now. The cramps in her legs are better, and so is the gall bladder – in the last 14 days these problems did not exist for her. The bloating is reduced, so is constipation, and the fear of driving her car has left her completely. However, the main thing is that from the beginning, since she started to take the preparation from prana (she reached the potency of

7.5 liters), she has, as she had put it with smile, the feeling of "having her brain taken out from head". She thinks a lot less. We talked about it for a while, and had concluded that it was this excessive and useless thinking that was her main problem. With less thinking there was less suffering. Otherwise at work (she has an intellectually demanding job), she manages to be as effective as before.

It is important not to think – for instance the prerequisite for Buddhist meditation is chasing away all the thoughts, and not everyone can do that. However, people on autopathic treatment have often noticed that things that happen around them, or that they themselves are doing, had begun to happen sort of automatically, without that great mental effort they used to have to spend. After a preparation from the information of the seventh chakra, many people told me that they feel happy once again. That they have feelings like in childhood. That things suddenly appear to be simple, as if happening on their own. I am sure that this exaggerated thinking, which we are being led to from the first year in school, and of which we sometimes become victims, is only a cheap substitute for something more profound. It is a substitute for a quality connection with the Universe.

When the connection goes wrong, we feel bad, crouching in the corner. Thoughts fly uncontrolled through our head, they do anything they want with us, and we fall ill. To cure ourselves, we must repair the connection, and that can be done through autopathy. How does it happen?! Which theory does it follow?! Why could ordinary water provide a cure?! Unnecessary questions. It certainly defies reason. Particularly the one of school, with a pigeonholed category, and the thoughts associated with it. Their possibilities are very much limited. Look around yourself, at how many rational people are so deeply unhappy. Then remember the moments when you were happy. I bet you that it was at the moments when you were free from the reason and thoughts you did not need at all.

Acute problems

A holistic autopathic treatment helps to handle even acute problems, such as sudden fevers of children and adults; there is good experience with this. The rules of tuning-up holistically apply here, the same as with chronic disease cases. In this correlation, let's recall Hering's Law of holistic healing, which says: "The symptoms are being cured in the reverse order to how they appeared." And this also applies for example to acute influenza, fevers, tiredness, painful joints, head colds and coughs. These arrays of symptoms have, from the point of long-term holistic developments, all appeared the most recently. Therefore these symptoms would be cured at first. *But, when the stimulated life force deals with the acute problem, it will not stop and it would begin to solve the chronic problems of that person's body and mind,* for instance his or her inclination towards frequent febrile illnesses. We have repeatedly been witnessing how, after a cured influenza, there followed an unusually long period without flu, and gone also were other problems such as headaches or rashes, or something else that person repeatedly or permanently suffered from. The AP made of saliva/breath or prana might be useful here.

The three parameters of treatment are to be set the same way as with chronic problems – *even acute disease is a sign of an overall state of being out-of-tune towards the reception of life force.*

Fever, P5 24 liters

It was a day before Christmas when the mother of an eleven-year-old boy rang me, saying that he has a fever. Even in the morning he was playing sports, but by noon he became languid, feeling cold. By the evening he was in bed, with a red face, feeling exhausted, and with a temperature of 39°C/102.2°F. I drove there with a bottle and instructed them that the boy himself should make the **Prana 5** preparation in the bathroom, letting the AB stand under the filter for **12 minutes (24 liters)**. The boy managed easily – he has been on autopathy since birth, taking it usually for something acute that passes quickly, otherwise he is completely healthy. The previous potency he had two months before this was 10 minutes, 20 liters.

A few minutes after the application of P5 he had his temperature measured, and it was already lower by a degree. Two hours later his mother sent me a text massage saying that he was down to 37.3°C/99.1°F. The next morning he had 36.6°C/97.9°F and no sign of illness.

Thus the fever was again the signal of an overall relapse, and the end of the effectiveness of the previous dose of autopathy, and a request for more in a higher potency.

Then he left for a summer camp, where an outbreak of quinsy happened to occur. Two days after returning he got a sore throat, no temperature, and it went away to the next day by itself – his organism quickly coped with it. Still, after the problem subsided his mother gave him, without a consultation and apparently unnecessarily, **P5, 10 minutes**, just to be sure. Since then, the boy has been healthy for the following year. By the way, the boy is continuously successful at school and is highly placed in sporting competitions. He can sit comfortably in the full lotus position, even though no one had ever taught him to do that.

With acute problems, the potency should always be set up in accordance to the overall vitality the person had before coming down with acute illness. With people who have been using autopathy for a long time, our point of departure is the previous functional potency, which we repeat or slightly increase.

If there are any significant signs of inflammation (diarrhea, head cold, cough, etc.) present with the acute feverish illness, it is appropriate to use SBB. There are, however, occasions for acute use of autopathy, other than influenzas.

First aid, box jellyfish

A sixty-five-year-old man was swimming in the tropical sea, and when he got out of water he got a strong headache, which he normally never had. The pain was getting worse. He noticed that on his heel he had a painless bloody gash that was fresh and deep. Because he had once been stung by a jellyfish, he could see the similarity. He also knew that in these seas one of the most poisonous creatures of all can be found, which out of all water creatures is responsible for the most of people dying – the box jellyfish. At a nearby stall he bought *a bottle of plain spring water, he spat into the cap, poured water to overflowing, poured out, and poured in more water and it poured out (the droplets on cap's walls carried the information).* He did this twenty times. *He poured the last filled cap on his forehead above the eyebrows. This was the so-called Korsakov's homeopathic dilution,* which I have described in all my books on autopathy as a method of first aid. It has turned out less effective (and in long-term treatment always non-effective) with treatment of chronic diseases, but with acute conditions it could sometimes bring about instant relief and aid, because an unused bottle of water is usually on hand. The strong headache after the sting by a box jellyfish (later he found out on the Internet that it was exactly that) went away in a few minutes. He went into the hotel, where he made a preparation of Prana 5 in an autopathy bottle, with 15 liters, which was his usual potency that he has used before. *On the Internet you can read the warning that in cases of stinging by box jellyfish, medical treatment is essential, and hospitalization lasts at least a week.* Seniors or young children in particular can die if stung by box jellyfish. The man (a senior) nevertheless went to dinner instead, and apart from a slight stinging sensation (like from an ordinary jellyfish) echoing for a few days, he had no more problems. He was left with a scar on his heel.

This is not to say that you should not seek a medical help in any health situation (whether you use autopathy or not). **With acute illnesses and sudden health emergencies of any kind, we should take into account the doctors' opinion, and appropriate** *conventional treatment.* Sometimes so-called acute symptoms, of which there are many, could in reality mean the worsening of a chronic pathology, involving for example the inner organs, and not only a "viral infection". It could also be a manifestation of "side effects" *from* taking medication, drugs, etc. Nevertheless, during the course of conventional medical treatment (or at any other time), autopathy can be used as a spiritual complementary method. In a person who suddenly and inexplicably gets a high temperature or a similar acute symptom, and who has been under autopathic influence due to chronic illness, it could also be a cleansing, detoxification curing crisis – if there were lasting, deeper, autopathically-achieved improvements of the chronic illness. Then it might be prudent waiting with autopathy until the next day. Only if the situation has not significantly improved within twenty-four hours, it is possible to repeat the same potency that was used before, and that has brought some beneficial result in the mind or body, or which the person takes regularly, but shortening the interval between applications. On our website there is an article on autopathy and small burn marks, describing the case of a lady treating a chronic illness with autopathy, who burnt her hand while ironing, and how she shortened the interval of applications. She took her usual AP immediately, and the injury healed quickly, with the pain subsiding. There are even some photos online ("Autopathy and small burns" at www.autopathy.com).

Acute problem, change of method of preparation from P2 to SB and SBB

Sometimes with an acute problem it is advisable to change the method of making the AP. A lady eighty-seven years old, who was treated autopathically for sixteen years. She is vital, looks after a large garden with her husband, and often looks after grandchildren and great grandchildren. She also spends a lot of time in the kitchen – her traditional meals are reinforced by her own grown vegetables, home-baked bread, home-bred rabbits or eggs are popular as well, and she is the central entity of a large family. She weights over 100kg/220lbs. Last spring and summer she was taking P2, two minutes flow (4 liters) – she has water well – once every 14 days, and she was conspicuously happy, with her main problems connected with being so overweight. A detailed description of her case could, due to such long-term observation, fill many pages. It is only worth mentioning that over those sixteen years she had never stayed in hospital, while before this, she did. Occasionally she goes to the doctor for a check-up, but nothing serious was ever found. In August last year, however, she got strange and strong abdominal pains with a sense of fullness; the pain was getting worse. The doctor did not know what the problem is, so sent her to do CT tests. In this acute state we had changed the autopathy to BB, **two minutes** (4 liters), which she took daily. The pain went away in a few days. After changing to **2.5 minutes (5 liters) SBB daily**, the sense of being full had gone too. The CT tests that were only done after that did not show any pathological find. During this treatment she has also lost 10kg/22lbs, and for the first time in decades went under 100kg/220lbs. She continues on SBB, 2.5 minutes, once a week: she is active, merry, and for her age certainly healthy. By the way, as always she smokes three or four cigarettes a day, but she does not smoke for a day before applying AP.

Part Three

MISTAKES

Possible mistakes that could be made while practicing autopathy, and how to avoid them

To get better, in the context of autopathy, we must do everything within the rules that have been found out by observation during the sixteen years of it being practiced, as they have been described in books, on Autopathy.com, and in records of conferences. Mistakes, or breaches of rules, are hindering our progress. In extreme cases they even stop us, send us back for a while, or for a long time. But they also teach us. Through mistakes we can learn a lot.

The case full of mistakes: Twelve years of autopathic development

A young woman, in a rather stressful profession. Twelve years ago she came to see me, because in summer she could not breathe at night due to an irritant cough, which has happened four times. For years she had allergies in spring, later she had headaches and an aching back. During the consultation I had recommended an AP of **saliva, 6 liters, one-off** (the "wait and watch" system).

She did not come back, until five years later. She reported that she was absolutely fine for two years after the one-off application of the AP, without the previous problems. However, her asthma intermittently came back, for which she used a spray. The headaches also came back after two years. Often she had laryngitis, a cough, quinsy, and once a month mycosis before menses – all of this she muted with pills. The spring allergies had come back. Menses at the time of her visit were stronger and lasted a week; it was exhausting, her head and back were painful, and as she said "I couldn't think, I am useless". It starts three days before and goes on for three days afterwards, it hinders her at work and elsewhere; this is why she returned. I recommended: **6 liters, breath (no boiling), once a month.** *6 liters worked very well five years ago, this is why I had recommended it again.*

The mistake was made when two years after the application her problems came back, she had completely forgotten about the good old time-tested autopathy. Yet, when her health, in a state of disrepair for another three years, had begun to further erode her sense of life, she did remember after all. She probably wanted to have her state of health improved the conventional way and acted conventionally, but she saw that it simply was impossible.

Follow-up interview in two months: She said that she did autopathy only once (**an error**, it was recommended to be applied repeatedly), she sneezes in the morning, the symptoms during menses had improved by a half, there was no mycosis, her nose is not cogged, she has just passed by a linden tree and nothing – formerly she would have been sneezing. The dryness in her throat had gone, the nape of the neck was not sore at all, only once did she have a headache and it had gone by the evening, and it was less painful. The doctor had recently noticed the lobe on her thyroid gland could be a little enlarged, and had sent her for blood tests to have a hormone analysis – this result had not yet come back. I had recommended **6 liters, breath with boiling** (a new method at the time), once every three weeks.

She came to the next follow-up interview a year and four months later – **a fault**, she should have come in three or four months. Again, she did autopathy only once at the beginning, not repeatedly as advised, which was another **blunder**. The desire to be conventional was still very strong. Let's do autopathy and then forget about it. She said to me later that it was partially caused by her partner's stance, who did not understand autopathy and laughed at it, so that she would rather do it when he was not at home. Nonetheless, after a single application she was fine for more than a year. The suspicion her doctor previously had about the thyroid gland malfunction was not confirmed by the tests. Yet, light asthma appeared two months ago. It lasted for three weeks, mainly at night, and she slept very badly. It was in hot weather, during September that it settled down. Still, she is very tired and needs more sleep. She has a discharge and blocked ears. The recommendation was to increase dilution **from 6 to 9 and to 12 liters (BB), once at a time** ("wait and watch"), if the effectiveness of the previous application was waning.

Development in the following nine months only briefly: The discharges stopped immediately, the back pains had eased and later altogether disappeared, so did her shortness of breath. Blocked ears no longer bothered her, the tiredness was gone. Sometimes there were cold sores. She considered discontinuing the contraceptive pills, which she had used for a long time. In the very latest time however she had a strange feeling of restlessness, nervousness. In such cases I advise increasing the dilution to **13.5 liters, breath, and no more boiling.**

However, the nervousness and anxiety had become even more pronounced. She found herself under constant psychological strain and did not know why (here I add that she has a rather stressful profession). Increased the AP to **18 liters without boiling.** She makes her report this time after a week, and it is all bad news. She feels dizzy. The anxiety is still here. I had to think hard where the **mistake** was made: The problems had begun when I had rather unnecessarily increased the potency above 12 liters and **when the boiling stopped**, which obviously was the **main mistake.** *We should not leave the potency or the method of preparation, which work and move the case to the better.* The problems were now aggravated by the addition of a lasting headache. Recommended: **4.5 liters, breath with boiling** (BB) – a return to what had proved successful in the past. She slept throughout the next day, two days later the headaches were leaving and the anxiety disappeared very quickly. Restlessness was there only a couple of times and for a short while. A week later she was fully fit.

The next follow-up came nine months later: More than six months ago, for reasons she does not remember, she took a **one-off AP of 15 liters BB, and 14 days later 18 liters BB.** She had no problems worth mentioning, boils only occasionally and they left quickly. The last week, at the beginning of May, she occasionally felt a tickling in her throat and a clogged nose – sign of a retuning allergy? Repeat **18 liters BB.** Now she is beginning to suffer from her old allergy, which was not there at all last year. It has appeared three times, always at night. Recommendation: **AP of 4.5 liters, BB, once every three days, alternating with SB. After three weeks move onto 6 liters.**

Follow-up examination in two months: The problems left quickly, and for a month and a half she has had no problems. *Returning to the time-tested degree of dilution has paid off.* Yet, I had recommended increasing the dilution: **alternate 9 liters SB and BB once every 14 days.**

Follow-up in four months: After a month she stopped autopathy, because there was nothing wrong with her. This has more or less been the case till now. Advice: **No applications, wait and watch.**

In another three months: She is fine.

Two months later, while still OK, I advised her that in the case of a reappearance of tension, anxiety or fear, to take Prana 2, 4.5 liters, every four days, and report to me, otherwise do nothing: "wait and watch".

After this I had not seen her for more than a year and a half, while she was fine, but then she rang me that the sense of fear has been reappearing the past three weeks. Her spine and neck are hurting her. She has an unused bottle since last time, because she did no autopathy, and after such a long time without problems, she forgot about my advice on what she should do if the problems returned – a **slip-up.** First I recommended **6 liters HB**, but nothing had improved. A few days later **Prana 5** was recommended, following the procedure in the capitol (page 74), start on 1.5 liters and add 1.5 liters until she feels there is an improvement. She got to 4.5 liters and had not noticed any improvements. On the contrary, she feels dizzy and has headaches. I asked her what sort of water she used. I found out that she used a cheap one with a drinking water label. That is where the **fault** laid! Such chlorinated waters bottled from the common waterworks have not worked in autopathy. I know that from many people, who have had the same experience, and an instant rectification was in always choosing the correct water. This are labeled by manufacturers as "spring water" (not as "drinking" water) – and usually do not contain any additional chemical substances. I recommended using spring water without additives. In the three days after applying **4.5 liters** there was a significant improvement, then a small aggravation; she took **6 liters**, the psyche improved for three days; in 14 days' time she increased to **7.5 liters, Prana 5**. Some old physical problems came back, while the psyche was varyingly improving. **Recommendation: Repeat 7.5 liters if her psychological**

state worsened. Increase by another 1.5 liters, if there was no improvement.

Two months later she told me that the last time she repeated **7.5 liters Prana 5** was a month ago, since then she was okay. She gave the impression of being calm, balanced and she laughed – she had not looked this relaxed ever before. As to her appearance, she looked very young and fresh, I would have guessed she looked ten to fifteen years younger than she really was.

The last follow-up interview two and a half months later: She felt good, did not have to apply anything. She has plenty of energy – at work she has taken on more responsibilities. She recommends autopathy to other people. My advice: **Repeat Prana 5, 7.5 liters, but only if necessary.**

The summary: We always make some mistakes here and there. Errors in autopathy do not do any damage. They only mean that autopathy at the given moment cannot bring us the maximum of its potential benefit. However, if we learn from our mistakes, they become positive developmental stimuli, which help us to further move the boundaries of our knowledge about the workings of autopathy. The fundamental thing is realizing them – and rectifying them.

To the case of this woman, now in middle age, we might add that instead of spending the past twelve years with asthma, and later other chronic problems, the majority of that time she was healthy, only with short malfunctions corrected by autopathy. Taking into account the fact that 30% of our compatriots have allergies, it is a good news. The older this lady gets, the healthier and prettier she gets – more good news. The third good news: Let's not be afraid of making mistakes, because if we realize them, the rectification follows. Fourth good news: There exist books (three thus far) on the method. In them are summarized our experiences, they tell us how to proceed to make as few "mistakes" as possible, or to avoid them altogether.

Other possible mistakes that have been observed

Impatience in the treatment of chronic diseases, and from this often following **hasty changes** of strategy, potency, interval of application, method of preparation, without waiting for the adequate time (weeks) for evaluating the reaction. Chaos might arise, in which it is difficult to orientate ourselves, when we do not know which potency or which method of preparation worked the best, and what on the contrary worked less or not at all. *The solution is going back through records and using the method of preparation and the dilution that worked best in the past, and stay with them.*

Concentrating on a single problem, while not following the holistic development of body and mind. A beginner's error: the lingering conviction that diseases in people are separated and that they must be perceived and treated separately. Lack of a sense for wholeness. It can happen that a person only has one problem that appears to be unbearable, while the others may seem to be marginal. *To get over the top of the main problem, we must not lose sight of the whole, allow for Hering's Laws,* and not forget the fact that we always treat the central fault, which is the organism being out-of-tune with reception of the perfect, harmonizing and reviving life force. Diseases come about as a result of this culpability, and if that can be removed then there follows the state of strengthening and continuing health.

Short memory – autopathy has improved or solved some problems, and now it appears that it no longer is necessary. After a while it might be completely forgotten about, even though life's circumstances are continuing to be stressful, and this might eventually result in the problems returning. I recall one phone call, when a lady told me recently that once, seven years ago, she used to see me with a chronic cough, which had disappeared after the treatment, and she was now asking me which homeopathic remedy I had recommended then, because now, after seven years, it is coming back. I looked through my notes, and indeed, I had found her there. The chronic cough went away after one application of an autopathic preparation. When I told her, she could not immediately remember, and did not know what I am talking about... And then she sighed, "Oh, this, this autopathy ... I thought that you might recommend me some remedy." Sometimes of course, such a relapse, or return of a problem, can happen in a much shorter time. And then it happens that the person involved tries out a number of other methods, before humbly returning to autopathy, which has solved the same problem before. *Usually we select the same method of preparing the AP and the same potency, which have preceded the cure.*

Not keeping records of development, be it with self-treatment or when treating another person. In many long-lasting cases we meet with the situation when during the oncoming treatment the choice was not correct (see the recently described case of twelve years of treatment). For instance, after increasing the amount of water or changing the method of preparation, the effectiveness does not improve, or even drops down. Then it is necessary to look back and to see which potency and method of treatment worked best then.

Return to the time-tested, to whatever worked with that given person, but was prematurely abandoned. This kick starts another period of positive development. *Such a return is not possible without the records. Even imprecise records could raise uncertainty in dealing with a case.* It is very important to not only note the negative events, what is out of order, but also the *positive feelings and events,* the periods when all is in order – this is what tells you in which potency and method of preparation autopathy worked with the most intensity. That is what we can then return to. **Above all, it is appropriate for the person being treated to also keep those records.** Then it is a certainty then that nothing would not be lost, and if a consultant is being used, then the switch to self-treatment, or a change of consultant, is always possible. Keeping your own records also has the advantage that you can record your observations and feelings at the time when they are happening, which in retrospective facilitates an undistorted and accurate view of the case.

Not infrequently, and particularly at the beginning of the treatment, we meet with this strange phenomenon: *people do not realize at the follow-up interview five or six weeks later, that their condition has improved a great deal, that even a lot of their chronic problems have left them. It so happens that we have an extraordinary ability to forget the pains and negative phenomena if they have gone away.* Perhaps lax record keeping might help us to live our lives easier, but it is not helpful with making correct observations and evaluations of a case at the follow-up interview. This is when a well written and detailed recording of the initial interview is important to help with further treatment. If the records are slapdash, or do not exist at all, **it limits our abilities to successfully follow a case.** I have already included examples of this in the previous books, but here is another:

Nothing has changed, SB, SBB, P5

A lady, over fifty years old. She sleeps very badly, about three to four hours a night, and during the day she gets very tired. She works ten hours a day, and in her workplace she constantly takes on more work. It gets worse and worse, sometimes she does not sleep at all throughout the night. She wakes up with fear and feels anxiety – she thinks about various problems, while walking around the flat. She hates taking pills, does not have any. Nonetheless, she says it cannot go on like this, some solution has to be found, "or she'll go crazy". Heavy insomnia has been bothering her for twenty years. Since the previous year she also has problems with digestion, she is bloated, has flatulence and constipation. For thirty years she has been suffering from frequent inflammations of her nasopharynx, and she has antibiotics for that many times. Still, they do come. She has food addiction; she eats one chocolate bar a day and craves sweets. There is humming in her ears. During the morning, she has bloating around her eyes. She has had depression for a long time, day or night; nothing makes any sense, and nothing interests her, not even her work. A month ago she had begun self-treatment, after a course in Autopathy 1. In her self-treatment she took 3 liters S (saliva without boiling) once every four days. Her mood and her sleep had improved. Recently she had a sore throat, and when she boiled the preparation from saliva it improved, now only a head cold persists. She increased recently to 6 liters BB, but her sleep had gone worse to the previous level. The **mistake** was in not boiling the preparation from the beginning ("at the beginning of treatment we nearly always boil", such is the rule). Also, she wanted too much too quickly. Nevertheless, there were improvements, and they came in a short time during her self-treatment of chronic problems that had lasted decades. I had recommended to her: **SBB (saliva, breath boiled together), 6 liters, a week later 9 liters, and then 12 liters, once a week, until the follow-up interview.**
  Some people during the follow-ups express gratitude even for

small changes in their years-long ordeals. But there are others with a completely opposite orientation, and this lady belonged to this category. She came to the follow-up a month and a half later, and with a skeptical expression and tone of speech she clearly suggested that there will not be any celebrations over some success. During such moments, unpleasant thoughts usually run through the consultant's head about having incorrectly set up the potency or method of preparation... and that a lot of work lies ahead. And, indeed – the lady had reported: "Nothing's changed." "Nothing?" I had shaken my head with surprise. "I still sleep badly."

After this she assured me that she did everything as agreed upon the last time. I looked into my record from the initial interview, and asked her about her digestion. She had to admit that improvements were seen in both the bloating and the constipation. Last week the addiction to chocolate and the sweets had also gone (!!). But, and she has to stress that, the main thing for her is the sleep. She sleeps only four or five hours, and wakes up several times a night! I looked into the initial interview record, and found out the entry stating that she sleeps only three or four hours a night, so the time she is now sleeping is an hour longer. When I pointed out to this, she conceded that this might have been the case, but for instance last night she did not sleep very well at all. And then she remembered that a couple of days ago, over the weekend, she slept a total of eleven hours, something that has not happened to her for twenty years. Last week she was extremely tired, she was even thinking seriously about giving a notice at work, which still takes up ten hours of her day. But then she increased the potency to **12 liters SBB**, and the tiredness was gone. Since then she has not been tired. Also, since then she had neither depression nor anxiety, not at night, or during the day. Further during this follow-up interview she realized that the pressure on her chest, which she had forgotten to initially mention, is no longer there. Sometimes in her life her kidneys used to hurt, that happened recently and disappeared (old symptom reappearing). At work, while talking, she used to constantly cough a little, but she no longer does that. Her self-confidence is higher, she understands a lot of things, and is inventorying her life. Yesterday she solved one long-term relationship problem, simply got on the telephone and it was successful. She used to be sensitive to the cold, walking in a sweater at home. Now she walks in a t-shirt, for the past fortnight! The fault in her thermoregulation is gone! Her work interests her more, 3which was not the case for a long time; there even is some new enthusiasm, as it used to be. The most changes came after she had changed the old bottle for a new one. Before that she twice had the potency from 12 liters, but everything had moved a lot after that last one. *Such experiences with increased effectiveness after changing the bottle are quite common.*

A short summary: **Almost everything had improved,** *and in a significant way, after decades of adversity. Perhaps at the beginning of this follow-up interview that psychological mechanism was at work, which leads people while visiting surgeries to stress the problems, so as to invoke more solicitude. We meet with this sometimes even with autopathy, although primarily it is about self-treatment, and the majority of people by far do understand this. My recommendation was:* **Continue with 12 liters SBB once a week, or more often** *if there was some aggravation.*

The lesson: Never base your assessment on a short term of reference on the development, **or on a mere facial expression.** *During a follow-up interview always compare the current state of each symptom with that at the previous follow-up (follow-ups). If I did not have these accurate records, which would have been a serious mistake, I would not have been able to ask the right questions during the follow-up interview, and the case could have ended up in a blind alley.*

Still, the case, as often happens, continued further. A month later the lady reports to me that after the previous visit she had decided to **make SBB from 12 liters every two days.** She also realized that she made two mistakes: Once she forgot to spit and once breathe into the bottle. Mostly she got it right, though. Then she got some tingling in her throat and a slightly higher temperature. Also, the night before the follow-up she did not sleep well. She does not feel good, and wants to be excused from attending the course. I so interpreted it that the old symptom reappearing, the healing reaction, to autopathy continues. Most of the improvements from the previous time have held, there is no need to take any preparation. Recommendation: **Wait for two weeks (the interval of two days with 12 liters was too short), then continue with SBB 12 liters once a week.**

Follow-up in a month's time: *She has only one problem, she says, sometimes she sleeps badly,* only four or five hours. That is when she wakes up at night and ruminates over family or work problems. Mostly she sleeps six to seven hours, though. Recommended: **Prana 5, 6 liters, and wait, while improvements last, repeat or increase by 1.5 liters depending on feelings.** I had recommended 6 liters because of her vitality, which has been significantly improved after the previous AP.

14 days later the lady says, that two days after the application she slept one night only for three hours. But now she sleeps much better, even eight hours. The overall condition is much better, and she is not tired in the morning.

The moral: Multiple sufferings lasting decades could be solved, with the state of health returning in a mere four months, as in this case. The final switch to Prana 5 was a logical one, because the only remaining problem was in the lady's psyche. The return of sleep to normal was preceded by a short, insignificant worsening, the healing crisis. If I did not keep notes of every consultation, I probably would not have been able to help this lady.

Road to health, road to the unknown?

When seriously chronically ill patients get well, it could mean, from the societal and psychological point of view, an unusual and unexpected transformation, inwardly and outwardly. Thus some might find themselves in a new position, not only health-wise, but perhaps even socially – people might have respected their situation as a sick person, and did not expect much from them. And this could now be changing. To the better, yes, but to some it still represents a step into the unknown. Often important is the change in self-perception as well, for instance, that of being a victim. When this begins to change, when the body and mind are getting into order, a problem of self-identification might arise: Am I still the one who was the victim of so many problems, who had to constantly suffer, or am I now someone who is seeking and being creative in the new situation, designing an appropriate life program? A road into the unknown.

Naturally, with the removal of a chronic out-of-tune state, there has been a new space created for self-realization. Different people react differently to this. People with tendencies for overworking themselves would immediately take on more work. Those who love travelling would travel more. People, who like relaxing, would relax more. People who like to meditate, might meditate more. Sometimes, even those who never had such inclination would begin to meditate, prey or have any such activity. Higher degrees of the mind could be opening, realization of wider contexts, of possibilities for oneself. Life is asking to be heard. However, an excessive identification with the illness could also lead to abandoning the treatment at certain stages. Sometimes it is necessary to build up this changed attitude to the world and to one's own personality, and this could be a fastidious process.

The case arising questions, BB

A lady, about sixty. She has polyneuropathy, resulting in strange feelings in her legs. It is hard to walk for her, a maximum of about half a mile, and she drags her left leg behind, even though to her surprise her doctor says that tests show her right leg being worse. Her face blushes repeatedly, in fall and in spring, and she always has antibiotics for it. Her joints hurt – hands, elbows and knees – she has headaches and a sore back, has diabetes and for twenty years she has been having insulin, now four times a day, and still has a higher level of sugar around 10 mmol/L, but sometimes as high as 15. A few years ago they found borreliosis – the vessels on her legs were clogging, and she had an operation with bypasses. Six months ago she had a stroke, could not speak or write her name, and stayed in hospital. Since that time she has speech difficulties, and signing her name still presents a problem. Long-term she has been taking ten different medications a day, plus some for acute problems. I had recommended **BB, 1.5 liters, once every two days, for three weeks, then increasing to 2 liters once a week, then 3 liters once a week.**

I had recommended breath with boiling because there was a fault in the vascular system; there were other (basically auto-immune) problems, painful joints and back. I chose to cautiously increase the potency from 1.5 liters because the vitality was low at the beginning.

Since then she had two follow-up interviews, always after about a month and a half. Even the first time she told me that the pains in the hands have gone, she walks much better, her back no longer hurts, and previously after sitting down each time she had to stretch, and it was painful, but that is no longer the case. With the polyneuropathy there was a difference – she felt it before the treatment above the knee as a clenched stocking, and now it descended below the knee, as per Hering's Law of "from up, down". Before autopathy her left leg at hip would buckle, but that had gone after 14 days of applying the AP. She was still on 1.5 liters. Recommendation: **Continue with 2 liters, BB, once a week, if need be increase to 3 liters – up to 3.5 liters, if there is lesser effectiveness.**

The second follow-up interview: Before the end of using her autopathy bottle for three months, some of the already removed symptoms came back – the joints were painful and the leg was harder to bend. **As soon as she changed the bottle for a new one, it was quickly beginning to improve** (a phenomenon sometimes observed, mainly in the third month of applying the same AP). She increased the amount of water to 3.5 liters and shortened the interval to every second day. She feels very good. There were no problems with her speech.

The last follow-up was over the phone. Out of curiosity I had rung her myself, exactly half a year after the beginning of therapy. The usual blushes were not there that fall, the improvements from the previous follow-ups have either lasted or even deepened, the tiredness was not there. She keeps taking the ten kinds of medication daily, the same as before autopathy – and autopathy in addition to that. A significant improvement in health thus came after less than six months! She did not come to see me anymore.

The case presents a lot of questions: How is it possible that it progressed so quickly? Even with the well above average number of chemical substances that she took long-term? A possible answer: A hidden state of soul and body, karma, merit. It is also proof that chemical substances and autopathy do not interfere with each other. The medications that she has been taking for a long time have their effect only on the body's level; autopathy has directly influenced only the fine-mater part of the person, reception of prana. Seldom have I seen such a fast cure of serious conditions, and that includes people who have not been taking any chemical substances.

Why did she not come any more, even after two years? One possible answer: She looks for the way of psychologically and

156

socially dealing with the improved state of health. Does she still do autopathy? Who knows? More likely, yes. At the last follow-up I had advised her to go up to 4.5 liters BB if necessary in case of lesser effectiveness – it is possible that she is still there. Maybe she does not consult with me, because there is no reason for it? In addition, her relative went through the courses of autopathy and now she is advising her, which would be absolutely logical. But I am sure that psychological and social adjustments with such a fast change may not be simple. Not only for her, but perhaps also for the doctors, who were confronted with such unexpected and unexplainable metamorphosis? Would they react by changing their attitude to the case? Or would everything – after a six months' pause – begin to return to the original state? It is a pity that I am not and possibly never will be, able to answer these questions.

It is good if after a significant improvement, or solution to his or her problems, the client keeps visiting the consultant. The inner tendency towards illness (being out-of-tune) may not be completely removed, and it is useful further and perhaps in a slightly higher potency, and in larger intervals, to repeat the AP, if only to prevent the possibility of a relapse.

(Un)freedom of thought

I have to say that I have met (rarely) with people, who stopped using autopathy, because for them the adaptation to new ways of perceiving their own self, their health, and the world, was too difficult. For instance, including the admission that after having experienced autopathy, that matter is subjected to fine-matter (in European and homeopathic tradition it is called "spiritual") influences. Educational systems and the media pump into us from childhood the materialistic view of mankind, which for some people and for some states, principally for theirs health systems, have by the beginning of the 20th century already become the norm, or even a compulsory religion. At the same time, primality of the fine sphere over matter is to be found in the important line of European philosophy and science; it has been continually recognized, up to the present. To some people we could give the advice: read the works of Plato, Pythagoras, Plotinus, St. Hildegard, Comenius, Berkeley, Newton (not only the creator of law of gravity, but also an alchemist), Swedenborg, Blake, Hahmemann, Kant, Schopenhauer, Bergson, Jung, Husserl, and leaf through the books of other well-known and acknowledged personalities who have their bronze statues in city squares. Or read some of the recent works of contemporary biologist R. Shaldrake, or quantum physicist and philosopher of science B. d'Espagnat. To be subordinated to power structures in concerns of freedom of thought is a **mistake**. It could even impede us on our way to gaining health.

Yet, autopathy has a chance. A survey in 2005 on the belief in the *existence of spirit and life force* by the Statistical Office of European Commission[1] found that Sweden was in front with 53% of citizens, followed by the Czechia with 50%, and Denmark was next with 49%. In many other countries belonging to the EU, the situation is similar. At another place of the same

---

[1]   http://ec.europa.eu/public_opinion/archives/ebs/ebs_225_report_en.pdf

survey on public opinions an even higher percentage of Europeans keeping this view is mentioned: 77%.

Part Four

PLANTS AND ANIMALS

Plants

A number of people have had positive experiences with healing plants, and let us know about them. I have already mentioned this in my previous books. In the meantime, these experiences have expanded, and it has again been confirmed that plants, be it in the garden or in fields, or elsewhere, can profit from autopathy. All things that are alive are also connected to the Universal Source, from which they draw information and power for their growth. Treatment is usually done using the Korsakov method (page 135, Acute use), because, **unlike people or animals, plants need very low potencies 6–12 C** (6–12 times pour water in and out the lid), singularly, as it appears, up to 30 C. Higher potencies have not been effective. Sometimes applying the potency once-off is enough and it could even have a long-term effect. It can be made from pulped sick leaves, from the needles, or any other green part, for instance from a bud. A sterile medicine dropper can be used, with a lid from a bottle of spring water. A clean glass vessel might be even better. A facial mask and latex gloves would be desirable.

We spread the sample from the plant a bit, stir, pour water to slightly overflow, we pour the content of the last lid into a can (or a sprayer) – which had not held any chemicals, and water the leaves, stem and roots. Naturally, this could be done even with a healthy plant, observing any effects on growth or quality of fruit. If we do it at the beginning of a season, we could get some results even in the same year. I concentrate on treating people, which I consider to be the most important, and have little experience in this area. Therefore I rather think of treating plants in terms of an experiment. However, during the autopathic courses a lot of people have reported successes – even in cases where from the conventional point of view there should not have been any expected, and also some articles by growers on www.autopathy. com are about successful results. With parasitizes we can boil the gathered substance before diluting (the AB could be a solution, but only using 0.3 – 0.5 liters of water).

Instead of chaffing the plant in water, we could also tilt down a live leaf into a vessel with water, soak it there for about half an hour, and then make the potency.

There are more articles about people's experiences with healing plants on www.autopathy.com. **To find full article put its name or a keyword to the search window on the first page.**

„*Application of autopathy against American gooseberry mildew*" by Tamara Krejcarova describes how she cured her gooseberry from the incurable disease powdery mildew. There are even photographs of the streaky berries before the treatment and beautiful ones after. I can imagine how useful autopathy might be to ecological agriculture.

The article "*Herbs and autopathy*" by Blanka Masarikova is about several kinds of herbs – mint, nasturtium, spear saltbush and others – attacked by a tiny worm, and how the problem was solved by autopathy.

Another interesting article is by Ludmila Vranova, which was originally a contribution to the 3rd Conference on Autopathy, "*Autopathic self-treatment and treatment of plants*". In the article, the following paragraph can be found:

"The idea that I can manage everything through autopathy did not leave me; instead it got stronger when I began to treat my plants, and had been able to verify its effect on roses, which had been restored from their infested and twisted leaves. From the state of vegetating, they have reached the state of 'health', have sprang new buds and brought them to flowering, while even the leaves were smooth and shiny. I had similar good experiences with languishing passion fruit, and with rosemary attacked by mildew, etc."

I presume that the author had used the methods of preparation and choice of potency, which I mentioned earlier in this chapter, because otherwise she did not specify.

Animals

When choosing the potency with the animals, we follow the same rules of "according to vitality" as we do with people. The potency and the method of making AP are the same. Also the same are the criteria for selecting the method of preparation. Saliva can be used for making the potency, which is collected with a sterile dropper (the treating person wears a facial mask and uses latex gloves). One lady, as I have already mentioned, cured her dog's chronic illness by having the AB in a plastic wrapper cooled outside the window, and waited till the dog breathed in. She held his mouth closed so that he had to breathe out through his nostrils, by which she held the bottle's funnel. She immediately washed the dew that formed into the vortex chamber, and the dilution by water followed instantly (the water could also be boiled beforehand). The resultant potency made of 6 liters of water was dripped onto the dog's nose. Thus she achieved a cure of his chronic problem. **Such contactless gathering of information through precipitation of breath on the cold surface of the funnel can also be used on a sleeping child, or a person who cannot participate.** A number of people have already done it. Another attendee at a course also did this with her cows.

A lady made a Prana 1 preparation for her dog. She held the water in a tilted AB a few centimeters above the dog's head near the end of its spine, made the potency, and dripped it onto the dog's snout. She used 1.2 liters of water, and applied daily. The old dog stopped its chronic vomiting and its mood improved. Whenever the dog saw her lady getting ready for making preparation, it distinctively expressed joy. With animals, the potency is determined under the same criteria as with people (with one caveat – the highest potencies have not yet been tested by anyone).

Liba Vankova writes in her article on Autopathy.com titled "*The New Year's Eve Theme*", about how she treated her bitch for panicked fear of explosions, fire crackers, and thunderstorms.

These events made her dog reluctant to go outside and made her so fearful that the sudden sound of a fire cracker brought about a bout of stiffness with twitches and shaking in her like in an epileptic seizure. The author of the article was inspired by my essay on making an AP from Prana 5. "I had used autopathy when the dog was restful; I waited till it laid down to sleep on its side. I poured a little water into the AP bottle, held it about 5–10 centimeters (2–4 inches) above the dog's head for about two minutes, approximately in the line of the spine, though I moved the bottle a little in all directions. After diluting with the required amount of water, I held the vessel again above the seventh chakra for about 30 seconds. Afterwards I moved in intervals of 30 seconds, always in the distance of about 3–5cm/1.2–2" from the surface of the body, first along the back of the dog..." She moved the preparation over the same chakras on the other side of the body, along the belly. After Mrs Vankova had applied the preparation in potencies from 1.5 liters and following this in 3 liters, in a matter of days the dog had lost her fear, and shortly before New Year's Eve, when the firecrackers were a regular occurrence, she displayed no fear or physical manifestations of such.

Veterinary practitioner Dr Jiri Stanek achieved the return of health in two ponies, suffering from allergic disease, *chronic obstruction of the lungs.* He had repeatedly applied the AP from breath. He says that after the autopathic treatment "The horses are capable of normal running, they do not get winded, enjoy their lives … bronchial tubes are penetrable, they can breathe perfectly..." This happened even in a hot summer, when they used to have the most problems. Also, inflammation subsided with another chronic disease in their hooves, which were also of allergic origin. He describes this in detail on a video made in the stable with both horses present: "*Chronic obstructive pulmonary disease in horses*". He used the already described technique of holding the funnel of the AB in front of the nostrils, bedewing the glass, and washing it into the vortex chamber, before dilution. The first week the horses were getting 1.5 liters daily, after this 6 liters twice a week for a month, then 6 liters once a month.

Another article is about successful cure of a guinea-pig. Gabriela Novakova: *"How a guinea pig brought my daughter to autopathy"*.

I also turn your attention to my article *"Autopathy also improves animal health"*, where I describe how I cured our own dog from a long-lasting chronic state, when a quantity of white phlegm was being discharged from its eyes and genitals. I used a potency made from saliva, 4 liters, one-off. The problem has not returned even years later.

Part Five

THE COMMON SHARING OF EXPERIENCE

The Conferences

Beginning with the year 2009, people practicing autopathy gather annually at the turn of January and February to share their experiences. They talk about what they managed to cure in the past year, what they had discovered, what caught their attention, which problems they had faced – and debate about it. It is a day-long meeting, in a large congress hall full of people. There have been ten such conferences so far. There are usually about sixteen to twenty presentation talks, one of which is mine. Prevalent are casuistic descriptions of cases about chronic incurable diseases covered by autopathy, often to their complete cure. From these cases sometimes unfolds the theoretical part, or generalization of the practical experience. The term "theoretical" here does not mean "speculative" or "hypothetical", which could be met with in the mainstream science, but it is always based on empiric real-life observations of what was recorded while

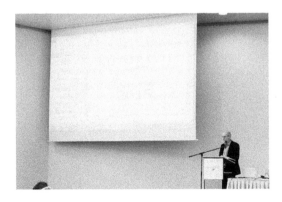

following the genuine cases. During conferences, a beautiful working and friendly atmosphere reigns, the participants realize very well that they are part of the creation and development of something that not only brings about a practical benefit, relief and return of health, but also new values, new meaning of life. Audio recordings from each conference exists on CD, about seven hours long (issued by the publishers Alternativa), which is available to the general public. So it is even now possible to study each of the conferences held thus far and be inspired by them. Apart from this, parts of the contributions are regularly published on www.autopathy.com, in text form.

I will mention some contributions, which I often recall when the talk is about conferences. There are the experiences of participants that inspired us all very much, and that brought a particularly large encouragement, and practical information even for my own consultancy activities. I will not include those that have previously appeared in my books. As there were already much more than a hundred reports (some lasting over an hour and some including descriptions of several cases of treatment), I cannot say that any of them would not be seminal, it has to be only a random selection. Their common theme is treating factual cases of chronic (formerly "incurable") diseases, and their so-called case history. Substantial parts of them have

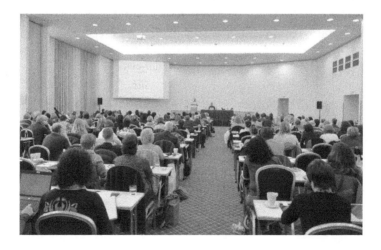

one thing in common; they are cases of people who otherwise have had – taking into account their occupations – no special prerequisite for healing. It was their own dismal situation, or of their near ones, and the unsuccessfulness of the previous methods of treatment, which made them begin to use autopathy for self-treatment. And naturally, of compassion – this basic and specifically human characteristic and motivation, which lead them to helping others. *Autopathy is a way of compassion with other sufferers.* However, even if we only treat ourselves, we still help others, because we radiate the vibrations of better health around us. Even the state of being healthy can be, as it appears, infectious!

Rheumatoid arthritis

In 2015, with agility, a man of stout figure and over sixty mounted the steps to the high podium at the congress hall of the hotel Pyramida in Prague, and introduced himself as Josef Jermar, the economist: "*Healing family members and friends, cancer*".

He told us his own story: In 2008 he fell ill with rheumatoid arthritis. All his joints hurt him; he could walk only with difficulty and on crutches. Merely combing his hair was an ordeal for him. Apart from the physical disability, he was also affected psychologically, and besides corticoids and analgesics he was also on anti-depressives. His condition was worsening; he stayed in hospital several times, any improvements were only temporary. In addition came heart disease.

He eventually found an autopathy consultant, who had recommended "*... autopathy, **saliva diluted with 1.5 liters of water, once a day**. Gradually I increased the saliva dilution to 3 and 4.5 liters. I endeavored to help myself. After going through the courses, I gradually increased to **6 liters** twice a week, originally the saliva boiled, and later with constant increases – now the boiled breath up **to 18 liters once a week**. After a year of autopathy I could put away the crutches, while still taking the corticoids. My weight increased, I blamed the lack of movement and*

169

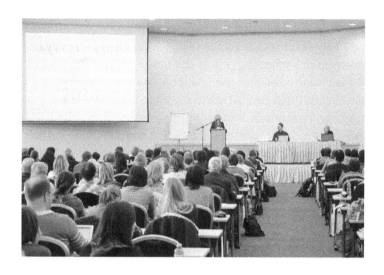

the corticoids. When walking, I was still not stable, I used a stick. Another year of treatment went by. Before Christmas 2014 I went to a test with a rheumatologist. The blood tests were good – all negative. Nowadays I use the stick only for longer walks and for surety. I use autopathy only for acute pains in my knee, hurt in an accident – the **boiled breath in 5 liters dilution** *– intuitively. Once is enough, the pain is gone."*

Quality of life

Other than this, in another part of his discourse Mr Jermar describes how he managed to improve the quality of life of his friend, who two years before this conference was in a late stage of liver cancer, and after the conventional treatment had a prognosis of three or four months to live. Gradually, the cancerous tumors got substantially smaller, during the treatment the diseased man was returning to various activities that he was previously unable to achieve. His life had gained quality, and got substantially longer, when on Mr Jermar's advice he began to use autopathy, first **SB, and BB, later SBB,** usually in frequently repeated applications, and increasing potencies, **from**

1.5 liters, up to 12 liters. Later he used **saliva and breath in one preparation without boiling**, from **18 liters twice daily up to 25 liters once a week.** Gradually the main tumor had got smaller, from 6x4cm/2.4x1.6" down to a third of its original size. Mr Jermar had also noticed that after two months of applying APs the reaction is lessening, so he was changing the bottle more often than is recommended on average. A year after this conference he told me that the man concerned was, according to the doctors, the longest living patient with such diagnosis that they had seen. Two years after the conference I had heard that the patient had died.

In other parts of his contribution, Mr Jermar described how he treated other people around him. He is a nice example of how, once a person tries autopathy on himself or herself, they also begin to treat others. The surroundings of such a person become a better place to live in.

Lowering of PSA to norm

1. One of the unforgettable reports at the 2013 conference was that of Stepan Robek. Its title on www.autopathy.com is "*Lowering of PSA to norm*". The author describes his own experience of autopathic treatment for a serious illness. I recommend reading it in its entirety. It is one of the few works concerning the feelings of a person who, out of the blue, was told by doctors that he has cancer. He found information on autopathy in my article in a magazine *on alternative healing*. He bought the book and a bottle, went to the course, and got to work. He never undertook any of the orthodox procedures that, according to the doctors, awaited him. Here are a few excerpts from the relatively long text. "Considering my diagnosis and my age over sixty years, I intended to begin with the potency 40 C (1 liter), but on account of my good vitality, I had decided to go for **60 C (1.5 liters). For the first month daily, saliva boiled, the second month boiled breath** […] After two months, well adjusted, I went to the laboratory for test results that would

fulfill my expectations. An incredible delight filled my whole body when I looked at it, and only now my hands had begun to shake. The PSA value had dropped from 6.8 down to 1.28 (editors note: the normal value is up to 2.5).

"Twice I had, apart from this, used autopathy to ward away quinsy. Twice daily for two days applying **40 C saliva boiled** was enough [...] Autopathy became daily part of our life [...] Let me also tell you that after this cure I told my colleagues about my diagnosis and the treatment quite clearly and without embarrassment at the annual meeting of our company, and at the New Year Eve celebration of our canoeing and trekking club, attended by about 70 of my friends and acquaintances."

I would like to add to it that the role of autopathy in cases of malignity, cancer, and various serious diseases, I conceive in our contemporary social context as complementary, as a spiritual addition to the conventional health care. I do not want to create the wrong impression that autopathic harmonization of vital force is something simple, guaranteed, always successful. All depends on our karma, which we create ourselves. Autopathy may not happen to be at all successful! And, finally, let's remind ourselves that even we, who use autopathy, will one day die. Death is a natural part of life. However, in our culture it is unmentionable; any reference to it is taboo. People should think more of death, and include it in their day-to-day contemplations. They should strive to prevent serious illnesses, by a healthy way of life. We should take responsibility for our sufferings.

The case of schizophrenia, diabetes, polyneuropathy, incontinence and bad mood

Even at the first conference in January 2009 there were several contributions (all are available on CD) showing how autopathy can be a strong tool for health improvement. This is particularly in regard to self-treatment and health in the family. Most captivating to me that year was the report by Martin Sikner, describing how he treated a nearly sixty-year-old lady: She could barely walk, had heavy diabetes – injecting insulin four times daily. She had bad eyesight, blackened toes on her feet (due to diabetes) – the doctors were contemplating amputation. She had high blood pressure, pain under her ribs, painful legs, her coordination while walking was poor – sometimes her knees buckled, she suffered from incontinence, and was diagnosed with gout. She was also diagnosed with schizophrenia – she had delusions, heard voices, had suicidal tendencies, and most of the day she was weepy – all this for many years. She had polyneuropathy, and her feet were not reactive to touch. The treating person had asked himself two years earlier (in 2007) a question, which he repeated at the conference. With such a difficult case, is it possible to achieve anything? But he said to himself that he would try and got to work. He had never treated anyone before, but he accepted this as a challenge. He followed the procedures as described in my first book, where at this time the only description of making **a preparation was from saliva.**[1]

He had begun with the potency of **2 liters,** and gradually increased it while applying repeatedly. From the very beginning he could see improvements. He reported that now, after two years of autopathy, the lady is in good mood, she laughs, does not hear voices and communicated normally (the symptoms of schizophrenia are no longer there), her diabetes had improved to the point that "if she now takes something for diabetes, it is the lightest stuff that exists", and her glycaemia after meals "is even better than with a completely healthy person". She keeps no diet and even uses sugar, she used to have changes on the eye socket, but now her surprised doctor says they cannot find any. Her blood pressure is normal. The toes on her feet, destined for

---

[1] All other methods have appeared later, the next one being the application made of breath, first used with a lady with chronic back pains, where the application helped her to improve, but had not achieved a cure. After 10 liters breath without boiling, her back had stopped hurting her, and no longer presented a problem. This is how our techniques had been evolving – with especially difficult cases, where the thus far known ways of preparation did not bring about a full effect, and the Universe sent us something new! Somewhat later followed the preparation from saliva boiled, from boiled breath, and then from prana.

amputation, have healed. She walks better. The feeling in her legs is back – there obviously is no polyneuropathy. We do not know the interval of applications, it was not given, the author said that he followed my advice published somewhere: With the next application double the amount of water (I forgot about this advice I had in the turmoil of events, and I do not even know if it had not just come out of some theoretical consideration). **He always doubled the degree of dilution**, therefore he would have gone **from 80 C to 160 C, next to 300 C; then he would increase to 2,5 M (2,500 C), which he would have reached in 6 months; then 5M (5,000 C) and lastly, after two years of treatment the lady would have received 8,5 M (8,500 C = 200 liters,** or 100 minutes of flow under the filter). In this case none of the potencies were repeated. At present, Martin Sikner said at the conference that the lady is a "different person". Sometimes she has a chat with her psychiatrist, with the result that "all is fine". Now she reads without glasses, whereas she used to have glasses with a strength of two diopters. Her diabetologist is happy, saying that this lady is "his showpiece", and that he would like to take her to a show, and had recommended her a diet, which she does not follow. After autopathy, surprisingly, a wisdom tooth started to grow. The lady says: "I feel as if I'm thirty". I had met the author of this report at the seminar two years later, and he told me that the lady is still fine. So much for miracles not happening! *The return to health was facilitated here by the high potencies that the lady reached after a series of lower potencies. This is usually the recommended procedure, even though the increasing might not be done this quickly, and it is in fact a variation of the "wait and watch" system. If the previous lower potencies could not bring the case to the state of health – we increase. If the high potency from unboiled bodily information (breath, saliva, or both together in one preparation) is "overdone", nothing much would happen, but that there would not be the full, long-lasting healing effect. Then we return to the lower potency that worked well before. More on the use of higher potencies on page 185, "The power of high potency".*

Nevertheless, on a fine-matter scale our Source, from which the creative information that forms our body and mind, is the finest of all. Over time, we try to get near it by increasing the dilutions of the AP. It is only possible though to the level which the state of our body and mind would currently allow us and requires. It has nothing to do with the "higher" or "lower" level of spirituality of the involved person.

Epilepsy

In the 2015 conference Dr Martina Kormundova came with her contribution titled "Secondary epilepsy after enduring bacterial meningitides". A young man was suffering from epileptic seizures of the type G-M. "After each seizure for the rest of the day followed numbness and lassitude." The doctor had first recommended an AP from **unboiled breath 1 liter, twice a week**. The follow-up examination was in one month. During that period there were two seizures, but lighter ones, and after waking up the young man had recovered in four-five hours, instead of the usual entire day of lethargy. He continued with an AP **from unboiled breath twice a week, increased to 2 liters**. In the next month, only one seizure came, but the patient already returned to the normal state within two hours. "He felt overall more relaxed and described input of energy, higher vitality; psychologically he was calmer, not having such worries about the future." Recommended: **3 liters, breath without boiling, once a week**. Six weeks later he reported: "… he only had one light seizure the absence type and was in very good contentment, believing that he would be completely rid of epilepsy. Headaches are less frequent, lighter, overall he feels like being able to better think, contemplate." Recommendation this time was for **SB, 5 liters, once a week; and alternate with an AP of Prana 1, 3 liters, once a week – that is about every three days apply one of the above.**
Two months later the doctor learned that for almost a month's duration he had a head cold, a strong one at first, and after the application of AP from prana, he had a period of expressed

anger: "… he perceived how the suppressed emotions and fears are being released. For three days he was 'knocked off', then came a feeling of relief and calming down." And between the time of the two follow-ups he did not have in any epileptic seizures. The advice was to **continue with autopathy from prana once a week and the bottle thus far used for saliva to be used for auto-nosod, stool with boiling, once a week, 3 liters. Alternate.** Another follow-up: "There followed a great cleansing act, diarrhea, coughing phlegm from lungs – for about 14 days, but he perceived, felt himself to be lighter, as if everything was being released that had for years burdened and tied him up. No epileptic seizure for three months, which has never happened before". **Recommended**: Autopathy for the whole body[2] under a shower for one-to-two minutes, after this along the chakras down and up once or twice a week, according to how he feels. Follow-up if needed.

In another two and a half months it was again noted that he had no seizures (altogether for six months): "… he describes harmonization and calming down, headaches only after assertion, meets people more often, looks for a new job."

Dr Kormundova has had so many interesting contributions at our conferences, which she regularly attends, about how she helped people recover from often hopeless states that it could easily be made into a book. I do not know if she is contemplating to write it, but I hope that she does. Many of her outstanding descriptions of treating the untreatable can be found on Autopathy.com.

---

[2] Autopathy in shower – the bottle with water is first held in the seventh chakra, then successively moved down and then again up to the seventh chakra, from where the water is always allowed to trickle down the back. All the time (here for one-to-two minutes) the water pours from the shower into the bottle, with the information concurrently being made into potency. The discoverer of this method is my colleague Mr Jan Matyas, who reported on it during the autopathy courses where he teaches. I believe that it might function well only when an own non-chlorinated well is available, or a carbon filter for shower. Here this – still experimental – method of preparation was used only after the case was much improved by the previous autopathy.

How to lose a client

At the 6th conference Martina Ponocna described how she lost a client, who used to regularly come to her for massages, and who had Bekhterev's disease since she was fourteen – she was now thirty-six years old. She already had vertebrae fused together in her lower back with a reduced ability to move her head, and back pains – for which she took medication. Two months before the first "autopathic" visit a swelling appeared on the soles of her feet, moving to the insteps and toes. Another symptom of her disease was recurring inflammation of the iris in her eye, which she had for seventeen years, lately once a year. She had problems with sleeping and was tired. She also had recurrent irritable rashes on her back and on her fingers, with cracking skin. Mrs Ponocna advised her to try autopathy. She decided on a **preparation made of boiled breath**, mainly because she too once had inflammation of the iris and the hip joint, "... and the boiled breath from the nose had worked wonderfully!" She recommended **applying the AP twice a week, for the first six weeks from only 1 liter of water. "After that I slowly increased it to 2, 3, 4.5, 6, 8 and 10 liters – all once a week.** Then she followed with **12 and 15 liters** potencies once a week. We repeated each potency several times. At the end we got to **18 liters one-off."**

"After those 18 liters the lady was very happy. By then she was again sufficiently 'communicating' with her body, and she trusted it, so we had made an agreement that she would observe and when she realized that she needed to support it with a potency, she would repeat those previous 18 liters. After a time she reported to me that she repeated those 18 liters a couple of times, but that the intervals are growing shorter, so I had recommended her increasing to **23 liters**, again as a one-off, and wait. The lady told me that when she was making the recommended preparation, out of forgetfulness she had poured through **30 liters**. She nevertheless has been happy since that time, as everything is in order."

Mrs Ponocna in her report "*Bechterev's disease*" then goes back with more details of the course of treatment. "Even at the beginning of the treatment, after 1 liter the psychology had improved and the client said that she felt as if a weight was lifted from her heart." A large overall movement was recorded after 6 liters, particularly on the psychological side. "After 10 liters the swellings on her feet were completely gone, as were the back pains. She had entirely cut out the painkillers, and none since. On 15 liters she had a fever for the first time in her life, up to 39.7°C/103.5°F for three days. Otherwise she was without any significant problems. The eye inflammation had not come back since the beginning of the treatment, only a hint of it, as an old symptom reappearing. She takes no medication these days, is happy with her improved psychology, sleep and menstruation. Particularly so, however, with the overall relaxation of muscles on her back, shoulders and lower back, where the vertebrae are joined." At the end of her report, the author had (jokingly) added: "And unfortunately, she no longer comes to me for regular massages, because nothing hurts her anymore".

We lose our clients by giving their health back to them. This is how it should be.

Psoriasis, diabetes, high blood pressure

Miroslav Simunek in his contribution "*Cured (not only) psoriasis*" delivered a short description to the 2016 conference covering one year of holistic treatment for psoriasis on lady close to seventy years of age.

"She had the psoriasis for several months. It was the guttate psoriasis, which was covering practically all her body, except the face. The coin-sized patches were very itchy, especially at night. In sleep she would scratch and mark the skin. Every day she had blood marks on the bed and on her night gown. For several years she has had diabetes, injecting insulin several times a day, the values of glycaemia being 19–20 mmol/l, and blood pressure of around 180."

"Considering her poor condition, with the classical treatment not bringing up any improvement, she was willing to agree with anything that would offer her the slightest of hope." Recommended was **SB, 1 liter, daily.**

"Three days later she came to see me on her own to tell me with great delight that practically after the first application of AP the itching had stopped, and that after many months she can sleep, feeling 100% better."

"10 February 2015 – still without the itching, the patches are calm, without any peeling skin. The skin is peeling only in her hair."

A week later they increased **SB to 1.5 liters**, every second day. After five days in addition to the already achieved improvements, a sense of wellness came to her, and at the same time **saliva was also added to the breath (SBB) with an understanding that after a week she moves to 2 liters every three days.**

After two months of applying an AP Mr Simunek found out that "… after the psoriasis left, there were only spots a little bit darker than the surrounding skin, but without any further exposition. Only from hair she still combs out flakes of dry skin. The diabetes has a value of 6, she still injects insulin, but a lot less. The blood pressure is 140 over 80." The diabetes and blood pressure have thus come down toward the norm. Recommended continuing **SBB, 3 liters, once a week.**

Three months after the beginning of treatment (after the expiration of the AB) the lady had decided to end autopathic treatment in her still improved condition. 11 months after the beginning of treatment, the author describes the development thus in his report: "Her condition is still the same, she feels very good. She still combs out the flakes from her hair. It appears that there is an increased production of dandruff, though. Through some 'non-torture method' she managed to shed 10kg/22lbs."

There were many contributions at the conferences, and some of them described several cases of miraculous cures of "untreatable" diseases, even up to ten in one speech. Thus we have a large collection of proof that we can help ourselves, even when it looks pretty bad for us.

About some articles on Autopathy.com

Many authors have published contributions about their experiences with autopathy on this information center. **Publishing cases is an important part of our new field.** Here we show people that a way to health exists, even though they have thus far been brought up and kept under the conviction that they are suffering from an incurable disease, which will stay with them to their death. And if they make the decision, and if their good karma brings them to our method, they could get rid of their problems. They find out, above all, how to do it, how to individually determine our three parameters of autopathy. Where the obstacles are. The people who come to us, the consultants in autopathy, are exclusively those with so-called incurable problems. I have selected a couple of the contributions that follow at random.

Type II diabetes

An article by consultant Krystof Cehovsky "*Diabetes II: Return to health after first weeks of using autopathy*" shows how simple the 'unrealizable' journey to health could sometimes be. Let's wake up to the fact of what a burden to current civilization diabetes has become.

"A man aged about fifty came to me for a consultation in mid-May. Seven years ago he was diagnosed with type II diabetes – a reduced sensitivity of the bodily tissues to insulin. All the time since learning about the diagnosis by a doctor, he had been taking medication three times a day. The values of glycaemia have fluctuated between 7.4 and 11 (the high level of norm is 6). He has high blood pressure, for which he takes medication once a day prescribed by the doctor. For three years he has been having diarrhea every two months, lasting two or three days. He has erectile problems."

The consultant recommended the following system of application:

- Week 1: **Application from 1.5 liters daily, and alternate the methods from saliva boiled and boiled breath.**
- Week 2: **1.5 liters application, every second day, and alternate the methods of saliva boiled and boiled breath.**
- Week 3: **3 liters, every second day, and alternate methods between saliva boiled and boiled breath.**
- Week 4: **3 liters, twice a week, boiled breath.**
- Week 5: **4.5 liters, twice a week, boiled breath.**
- Week 6: **6 liters, once a week, boiled breath.**
- Week 7: **8 liters, once a week, boiled breath.**

The follow-up examination in two months showed that the levels of sugar in blood were stable at around 6. The doctor reduced the medication by 70%. The blood pressure was on normal, and the client takes no medication for it. There was no diarrhea and the client had not noticed any erection problems. He felt vital and fresh. He gave an impression of contentment. After this follow-up interview, Krystof recommended: Continue with the same dosage and use the method from **breath (no boiling) and each week increase the dilution by 1 liter. The period of application: once weekly.**

Till the next follow-up at the end of September, the man was on the potency of 16 liters, and reported that the improved condition from the previous period had stabilized. The diabetes medication was reduced by another one-third compared to the last follow-up. The problems he mentioned during the first consultation have not been present in any way.

Sometimes his knee hurts, or some other joint. The dosage until the next meeting was set as follows: **Take once every 14 days a preparation from unboiled breath, 18 liters, and rely on the feelings – in case of any problems, apply one-time only.**

Ulcerous colitis

Jan Matyas is my long-term colleague, teacher of autopathy, and one of the most experienced consultants. In 2012 he published an article "*Ulcerous colitis and autopathy*" about the treatment of a chronic inflammation of the large intestine, which is a heavy and limiting lifelong burden to bear for many people. He presents two cases. I cite from the second:

A young man, a sportsman, has diarrhea with blood six-to-ten times a day. It has lasted for two months. Mr Matyas recommended applying "... **boiled breath every second day from 3 liters, three times; from 4.5 liters three times; and from 6 liters two times**, after this he was to ring me. By the time of the follow-up interview, all was different. Even during the first week the diarrhea had stopped, and blood in his stool had disappeared; more prominent however became mycosis and swelling of lymphatic nodes, which had ceased after two days. During the second week of autopathy, a strong head cold and feeling of coldness came – both had left by the end of the second week. The client had begun to gain weight again, he did not have to watch what he eats, after a long time. The recommendation was to continue **every second day with 6 liters for three times, and 7.5 liters twice**, reduce to 4.5 liters (emotionally this potency suited him the best, I ask the clients which one makes them feel the best) after five days, still with boiled breath. In to the follow-up interview in five weeks' time came a healthy young man. The last two weeks he has been in full training again..."

Since then 17 months had passed, during which he takes autopathy approximately **once a month from 6–10 liters of unboiled breath**. After about a year, while under a lot of stress, he noticed the more frequent need to defecate (without diarrhea and blood), which was solved immediately by several applications of boiled preparation. All this time he has had no problems and takes no medication.

Parkinson's disease and MS

In 2010 Mrs Stanislava Polakova published an article called "*The Cases of Parkinson's Disease and Multiple Sclerosis*". Two cases are described there. The description of her case of Parkinson's disease spans four years. During the treatment she used autopathy from saliva (no boiling) in one-off applications. In those times, the AB was changed after each use, the application was always on a one-time basis. The case description is a wonderful demonstration of how a lot can be depicted in a few words.

A man, eighty-two years old. Initial state: Parkinson's disease in advanced stage, the man does not communicate, sits apathetically with a partially open mouth, strong shaking of his hands, sometimes the whole body. Loses weight, swollen lower limbs, takes a lot of medication.

First application May 2006 – **potency from saliva, 3 liters** of water in autopathy bottle – within a week the shaking had stopped, his mental condition is gradually returning, physical condition improved.

Up to now, **altogether eight applications of potency made from saliva were made. Second dose from 5 liters, each successive one increased by 1 liter, across a span of five-to-seven months, according to circumstances. Now – April 2010 – preparation made from 11 liters of water.**

Current state: The man lives a practically normal life – goes out shopping on his own, walks to visit his daughter (a total of 3km/1.8 miles), watches sport on television, gradually gained 10kg/22lbs. After a consultation with the doctor he takes only five tablets a day from the previous eighteen. He feels good.

Another case described in Stanislava Polakova's article is that of a woman suffering from **multiple sclerosis**.

A woman, slightly over fifty. The initial state: "… she moves with difficulty in her flat with the help of two crutches, lies down, has double vision (eye operation), bad sensitivity in hands (cannot hold a spoon), loss of memory, stuttering, head spinning – in the morning she has to take medication to be able to get up, depression."

After the first application in June 2006, **1.5 liters, saliva without boiling,** within three days strong headaches came and a tingling in her jaw, and then within six weeks a "very significant improvement of psychological condition". **After that, in about six-month intervals and always one-time, an AP from saliva was applied, with the growing potency: 1.5 liters, 3 liters, 4.5 liters, 9 liters and 10.5 liters.** There was a gradual improvement of motor ability in her hands, then improvements in walking – to the point when she walked at home without crutches and outside only with one stick, while her psychology and everything else remained at an improved level. Then she moved onto the potency from **breath without boiling, 12 liters,** after which the doctor cut out the corticoids. In six months **the same AP** was repeated. "The present state: The woman began to paint, uses the computer, found herself a job – two days a week … she bought herself an exercise bike, in winter she swept snow from the footpath, is in a good mood, happy. We will continue."

Excellent cases, simple, and with a clear gradual development towards the better, and occurring within otherwise "unimprovable" situations. In autopathy, three things are important that the consultant should possess, and they were in play here: a) talent, b) regular self-information of the development in autopathy – the transition to breath, which was at the time a new discovery, and which was followed by a marked improvement, c) compassion and a desire to be of help.

On www.autopathy.com there are many articles and descriptions of cases by various authors. There is a lot of material to study, and I recommend visiting it.

To be informed in regular way about the developments in this new field, it is useful to register at www.autopathy.com. People then receive email notifications about any newly published contributions, which usually moves the boundaries of our knowledge a little further.

Part Six

THE POWER OF HIGH POTENCY

High potencies from bodily information without boiling

If a case stops developing and some problems persist, or there is the tendency to slip back to already cured problems, or repeated applications of lower potencies are not bringing about any further development towards improvements, the basic rule is: **increase the potency!** *Up to 15 liters we can increase by 1.5 liters, but from there on the increase is by 3 liters. From 30 liters we increase by 10 liters, from 80 liters by a whole 20 liters.*

We can also make routine increases every now and again (see page 172, schizophrenia), and observe if there are any improvements. There is always the possibility of going back to the lower potency if it did not work and the effect was lesser than after the previous lower potency. We increase mainly when the suspicion is there that the case is stagnating, without developing further, and various, though perhaps even improved problems persist. This applies not only to the bodily information from saliva or breath, but also to the AP from prana. However, in the case of prana, there exists a not-so-well researched space above 60 liters, entering to which may not be so beneficial (the case of transition from P5 to unboiled breath, page 190).

Saliva or breath without boiling, high dilution

Allergy, eczema, headaches, S 45 liters

One of the early cases of autopathy, followed for eight years. A woman, about thirty, with a troublesome atopic eczema since babyhood, allergic to hay, mites, dust and pollen, and has hay fever during the pollen season. Once a week she has a strong headache, has to take a pill. Very sensitive to the cold.

We had begun with a one-off potency of about 100 C. Even on the second day the eczema got worse, turned red and itchier, and she felt like she had influenza. There was also a head-cold. She decided on her own to change the herbal cream for an other one without any claimed healing influence.

The eczema stayed about the same (like when she used the herbal creams), but the headaches were significantly improved! She no longer needed to take any painkillers – since the application of the preparation she had not had any. During the month and a half till the follow-up examination, a headache came only once, and it was mild. Advice: wait and watch.

Seven months since applying the preparation: On her face there has not been any eczema for about three months. Anyone can understand what such a cosmetic change would mean to a young woman! It still persists on her chest and neck, also on her elbows and knees. The itching has gone. She partially attributes this to seasonal improvement of eczema in summer months. She has no headaches at all. Also, she had no allergy during the pollen season, even though she took no medication!

Ten months after beginning of treatment. The eczema had begun to return, and the relapse has also been evident from sleeplessness, she wakes up more often. She made a **preparation from saliva from 5 liters of water (200 C)**. The insomnia had departed. Eczema persisted in an improved form, and in two months' time the headaches were returning. **10 liters** in the

AB had relatively quickly warded away all the problems, and a state of full health followed, such as she never experienced before. This lasted for a full year after a single application of the AP, after which the headaches came back, as did the insomnia. **She applied a one-off preparation of 30 liters, saliva without boiling,** and again there was a period of full health. She repeated the preparation in the same potency of **30 liters**, and in a year and a half she increased it to **45 liters.** At the follow-ups every six months we had nothing to talk about. Twice there was an attempt made to apply a lower potency because of trifles (such as dry skin), that did not work, and new applications in high potencies in the AB of 30 liters and later 45 liters quickly installed order again.

The moral: ***If the high potency worked well for us, repeat or increase it, never decrease, not even if the actual problem appears to be "small", and a "small" potency seems appropriate.*** *It is not so, repeat the same as the last time, or if the AP no longer does the work, increase. With potencies over 30 liters increase by 10 liters, with five minutes of flow through.*

Juvenile arthritis, B 200 liters

A prepubescent boy was brought by his mother, who said that he was diagnosed with juvenile arthritis by doctors. They told her that the disease is incurable. The joints in his limbs and his spine are hurting continuously for two years already, and he is taking medication for it. He suffers from headaches. He has facial tics, and speech impediments that cause him to stutter. It sometimes happens that he is unable to speak at all. He is tired. At the same time, he has problems falling asleep; he takes up to two hours before sleeping, particularly when he is tired. On occasions he was crying because of tiredness, but still could not sleep. He occasionally has strange bouts of inner aggression; he is afraid that he might do something bad, and he finds that difficult to suppress. He saw a neurologist because of this; they confirmed a finding during an EEG. He has clairvoyant states, having dreams that are fulfilled in reality. The mother relates how through the power of his mind he had set up a cell phone so that it showed a state of credit. He knows that his mother would call him, several minutes before it happens.

I gave him the autopathy bottle (again one of the early cases of autopathy) and recommended pouring 5 liters of water through it (the homeopathic potency of 200 C).

We always applied the AP from saliva as a one-off, with gradual increases of flow through over 18 minutes and 40 minutes, up to 100 minutes (200 liters), all this in irregular intervals. All was gradually improving, though in time there were small relapses. 200 liters S was applied twice, a year apart: there were always light headaches, but no other problems. The last dosage was 200 liters B (breath without boiling), and since then he no longer needed autopathy.

After the change to an AP from breath he became a healthy successful young man, in spite of the medical prognosis. **Breath without boiling applied in high potency appears to be the best method of making a preparation to finish the treatment.** I had met him a few years later by chance, and asked him how he was doing. He said that he had no problems. I asked him about his clairvoyance. That had stayed with him. Since the last application of AP breath from 200 liters, seven years had passed. Therefore the doctors' prognosis that his condition and the pains in his joints would only get worse, has not only been unfulfilled, but the opposite had happened – a state of long-lasting health.

The moral: *Even with the light signs of a relapse, the high potency should be used, one which had solved the previous problems. We always, even with the lighter, but lasting problems, tune-up the whole system of body and mind. The breath in the end had turned out to be more effective than saliva, the last high potency brought about high resilience and lasting health.* At the beginning of this autopathic treatment I would nowadays probably use a lower potency BB (currently the main method of preparation with the joint problems and back pains), before moving on to high potency, clear breath, no boiling. At the beginning, however, I knew only one method of preparation, from saliva. Here it is necessary to remind you the reader that the main advantage of our current practice is that we can select the best preparation from more possibilities, whatever has been most successful under similar circumstances, bringing the most direct and quickest effect – I call it **the optimization of selecting from three parameters** of treatment.

Pinworms, S, 60 liters

A university student, a strong young man who plays sports. He comes to tell me that "down there" in the bronchial tube he feels irritation that makes him cough, about once every hour. Spirometry found no problem, and according to it his lung capacity is twice the normal size. In his stool he finds pinworms, and he often has stomach pains. He feels the nasal tube is clogged, his forehead hurts in the morning, and he has quinsy. When staying in the cold, he has a sore throat. **AP of saliva with 30 minutes** of flow through under filter, 50 liters – almost 3 M, once-off. Follow-up interview in four months: The cough got lighter, then disappeared soon after application. The pinworms had gone from his stool, and the stomach pains stopped. His sleep improved – he falls asleep in two minutes and has no dreams. Psychologically he had improved – university exams are much easier, the nervousness is gone. He is completely healthy. He no longer came to see me. Let's remind ourselves: We can lose clients through their health being restored!

Why saliva and not breath? At the time I did not yet know about breath. **Why 3 M and not 1 M?** I knew the client for some time, he had a high vitality. *Nowadays I would perhaps begin with 1 M, 25 liters. With young people especially, into account come high potencies such as 1 M, and gradually increase to much higher (for instance 5 M – 74 minutes of flow through the AB, 8 M – 100 minutes of flow through, 10 M – 120 minutes flow through), in the late stages of treatment. They could nevertheless* *be used with no regard to age, taking into account the previous autopathic development.*

The case of chronic fear, increasing potency P5 and final transition to Prana 5 B, 74 liters

A charming university student tells me a sad story: Since early childhood she was always afraid of something, and got stressed even in ordinary situations. Since childhood she also has eczema. For five years she has had a food allergy, and the allergy tests always show high values. Three months ago she was getting ready for examinations, but was sleepy and felt that she cannot remember anything. Drinking coffee did not help. She had therefore begun drinking caffeine from injection ampoules. After this, she collapsed. In the evening, when laying down she had heart palpitations, felt that she cannot breathe in, had a tinkling in her hands and feet, high blood pressure, and huge anxiety. An ambulance took her to hospital. They had found nothing, but when she got back home, the same states followed day after day. She could not breathe, had heart burns and pressure in her head, and she could not sleep at night. A doctor gave her antidepressants, told her that she will be taking them for years; for some time she was taking them, it did not help. She had also seen a homeopath. She took three homeopathic remedies, but it was still bad. She has states of depression, she thinks about how to overcome it, being afraid that she has gone mad. She is scared of death, and thinks she will suffocate, wonders if it hurts, ponders over it – if death is the end of all... While studying, she has headaches, and takes painkillers. She is scared of going to sleep at night, feeling that she is no longer herself.

Recommended: **Prana 5, 6 liters**, applied as a one-off. If there was a good response, wait, if not, increase to 9 liters. Follow-up interview in six weeks. After the first application, nothing had changed. Three days later she had repeated it, with the same result. Four days later she therefore increased the AP to 9 liters. Even within two hours after this, she had begun to feel

190

unusually great, she says, and since then she psychologically had no problems. This had lasted for 10 days, then her fear came back. She immediately applied Prana 5, 9 liters. The excellent condition was renewed the next day. At the time of the follow-up interview she is without problems. She had always given the information to the seventh chakra. I advised her to repeat Prana 5, 9 liters in case of relapse, or as the case may be increase to 10.5 liters. 14 days after the follow-up came an inflammation of her urinary tract, which she had as a child in the fifth grade – an old symptom reappearing. She took antibiotics, and the fear returned (relapse), while the inflammation continued.

When she came back, I recommended **12 liters, Prana 5**. The fear was gone immediately after the application, within three days the inflammation had also gone away. She was taking the same potency every 14 days, because towards the end of the second week the anxiety began to reappear, which had always gone away after autopathy. She had a stressful period because examinations were near. Nevertheless, she says that for the first time she had gone through this exam time in peace. Three weeks before exams I had recommended **15 liters, Prana 5**. The same day after the follow-up, she had rang me with the good news that she had just seen the allergologist, and for the first time her tests came out negative. The values used to be high, she could not eat a tomato without having her lips swollen; now she eats a tomato, and nothing happens. At the next follow-up examination she told me she had repeated Prana 5, 15 liters, and had easily passed the exams. Long-term, she felt optimistic and without problems, perhaps for the first time in her life. Still, not long after this follow-up, she had again felt anxiety before sleeping, immediately responding with P5, with instant relief.

Three times she took 18 liters, but the third application was no longer effective, the anxiety disappeared within a day after application and she felt an improvement, but it only lasted five days. Then she increased to 20 liters and it again only worked for some days, and there came the relapse. Even a further increase to **Prana 5 30 liters** no longer had a long-time effect of psychological wellbeing. Later she had confessed that for

191

a limited time she had been trying out some other alternative therapies, which may have had reduced the effectiveness of autopathy. It was necessary to repeat more often, and recovery was not as certain as it was before.

That is when I recommended making **breath without boiling, 35 liters.** It had leveled up the condition, but examination time was on again, which was always an ordeal for her, so an improvement lasted only for days before the anxiety came back. After increasing to **breath without boiling, 40 liters** (20 minutes under the filter) all was quiet for three months, with no significant depression or need to apply an AP. After three months, the feeling of anxiety came back, so she increased to **42 liters breath without boiling.** Clear sailing for 14 days, then anxiety before going to sleep. She increased to **50 liters Prana 5.** Then it improved, after this she had a mild crisis for a few days. When I had advised her to wait – I call it the healing crisis, it can happen sometimes that old symptoms bubble up onto surface in a milder form, and then disappear. This had happened and she was okay for two months, but not in the perfect state, on account of final exams just happening. Recommended **54 liters, breath without boiling,** with no improvement, so several days later advised to take **60 liters, breath without boiling.**

*Here I remind the reader that **when some potency does not have an effect during the course of a gradual increase, we increase the potency further.***

This has helped. She repeated **breath without boiling** circa once a month, whenever she felt some need to apply the preparation, which was usually upon the return of her state of fear, even though only for an hour before going to sleep, and gradually she increased the dilution to **74 liters.** She did not need to go any farther, and she has been fine for the last six months.

When she tried to repeat the same potency, it never worked, but early increases always brought about the departure of the problems.

We had agreed on her continuing with the breath without boiling, always one-off application within the "wait and watch" system, and I had assured her about **74 liters (37 minutes of flow-through under a filter) not being the limit.** At the last contact we had, she already had the university degree. Her quality of life was much better than before autopathy, which has become a part of her lifestyle.

There are too many influences around us that bring about anxiety and depression. They cannot all be named, but the basic one is being out-of-tune as a result not receiving sufficiently the subtle information, the prana. We can feel it, and it terrifies us, we can sense that one way or another, things will turn out to be bad. We need to tune-up, to once again feel the harmony, self-confidence, health.

*From autopathy's point of view, the transition to **high potencies from breath without boiling** are usually recommended in the later stages of treatment, from 30 liters onwards, and with no regard to the original character of problems. Vitality, age, and other criteria are a decisive factor here. Important are the observed reactions to the lower potencies. When they cease to be effective, we increase them. But the opposite course of action is always possible: When the increased (high) potencies cease to be effective, we could again lower them. This always depends on feelings of the person being treated. There could be stages of development when high potencies are needed, which could be followed by stages when lower potencies would be more effective. For instance, with people around seventy years of age.*

The upper boundary of high potencies has not yet been discovered. I only wish to remind the reader that in homeopathy the high potencies codenamed CM (they are available in homeopathic pharmacies in England, India and Austria) have been proven effective, and in the reference literature often mentioned. This approximately would be the equivalent of having 2,500 liters of water flow through the autopathy bottle.

Making very high potencies

When making high potencies (over 30 liters), we can no longer do it with the plastic bottles of spring water. It is very useful to use a carbon filter for chlorine and other industrial pollution – there are many types on the market. **The best way is to have enough water from the filter flow into the AB so it is slightly overflowing (with a natural spring it could even be overflowing by a great amount), so that the surface is on level with the surplus water flowing over the edge.** In this situation, in 30 seconds the bottle lets through approximately 1 liter of water, which we control with a stopwatch. One minute = 2 liters, five minutes = 10 liters, 30 minutes = 60 liters, 100 minutes = 200 liters. Usually we do not need to hold the bottle, we can stand it with its bottom on a flat surface in a hand basin, etc. We could also make a holding device from wire, which would enable us to making the preparation on an uneven surface, round basin, in nature (on rocks), etc.

A holder that I used for making preparation by the natural spring well in the woods. It stabilizes the autopathy bottle on an uneven surface and keeps it in the upright position. When making

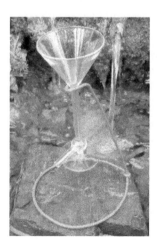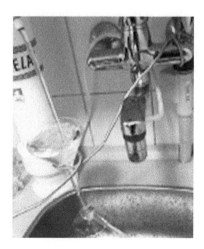

a high patency I do not need to hold it in hand for a long time. I used a 2-millimeter thick isolated copper wire with a hook on the end. The holder can be made with the help of pliers in about five minutes.

We let water flow into the bottle allowing it to overflow the funnel. Make sure that the bottle is not moving and that water flows through it steadily, and then we can read our favorite magazine while the potency is being made. It is advisable to stay near the bottle all the time, in case it moves at all, or the dilution is interrupted, etc. We could also attach it to the tap in the required position, as in this picture, which makes it safer, so that we could even go out to do our shopping. Such potencies usually are not applied often, and it can be many months till the next time we have to make potency again, under the "wait and watch" system.

Apart from that we could also use the filtered water for making drinks and food, as filtered water is tastier and of better quality, and it generally belongs to a healthy lifestyle.

Also suitable is making a preparation from a home water system, if it has its own non-chlorinated well as the source, or when we know that the public system is not chlorinated, which can usually be ascertained on the web pages of the water company (for instance in Germany, Switzerland, etc.). The presence of chlorine may not be detected by smell. Also added fluoride in water could be a problem, resolved by using carbon filter.

Some people, for instance at the conferences, have been describing unusual pleasant experiences of being at oneself with nature, energy flow, altered consciousness, extasy, etc., when they made high potencies from prana (up to 300 liters) by natural springs but also in their bathrooms.

Fear of the higher potencies

People sometimes, particularly with self-treatment, hesitate if they should go to the potencies higher than 30 liters with preparations made from saliva or breath. Even though they know that *when a previously successfully potency loses its effect after repeated applications **it must be increased**,* which is a basic rule in the process of *autopathic tuning-up.* Sometime there exists a fear of the higher potencies. It might be a fear of carrying heavy bottles of water. But it could also be fear of a change. A change from the state of disease to the state of health? From the change of being a victim to being an active participant, influencing not only one's own fate, but also the fates of others?

Sometimes it happens that people identify with the social role of a diseased person; even though they admit that they would like to be healthy, unconsciously they resist it. ***The disease itself is preventing them**, and it might even appoint some "reasonable" arguments as its helpers.* Whatever it is, let's realize that this fear does exist, so we may overcome it. If the potency really is overdone, for example, if in the third year of using autopathy I had made a preparation from 250 liters, just to find out what it would do), the positive effect was simply lesser and not as deep as if I had used the lower potency that would have been more appropriate. That is all. From the lesser effectiveness I could have found out that I am too high, and that I should decrease the amount of water. Sometimes a potency that is too high for a given case could result in a larger inflow of energy than the actual person can momentarily handle. Then the tension can be felt psychologically, not bringing about a sense of comfort. When the potency is lowered, it would sort itself in accordance to the appropriateness of the new potency. Finding the most suitable potency is generally the aim of our endeavors.

One participant of a course had told us of her case. Her eighty-year-old grandmother had a large brain tumor, and could no longer move, laying immobile in bed and having terrible bed sores. The lady had decided to treat those bed sores with a preparation made from saliva. She made it from 50 liters of water. At that moment I had jumped in: "Didn't I teach you that with low vitality we start with the potency from 1.5 liters?!" "Wait", said the lady calmly. "So I gave it to her, and she began to walk and the bed sores had healed. It had looked so hopeless, so I said to myself that there's nothing to lose."

There are exceptions that confirm the law, perhaps. It always is about karma. But this case certainly shows that fear of the high potencies is a prejudice that might sometimes prevent people from reaching the state of health, because they have stopped half way. *Practice has shown us that it is possible to divide people, from the point of view of an individually suitable potency, into two groups. Some people are more in need of lower potencies and their problems could be solved with AP from 1 to 15 liters of water. Most people appear to belong to this category. At the beginning of autopathy, all people belong here.* Another group of people, however, achieve the same goal only with high potencies, even though the preliminary lower potencies had helped them in the early stage of their development. Yet, the jump to the state of full health with them only happens after perhaps 30, 70, 200, or even more liters. None of us has their number written on their forehead, and presently, no machine could measure it. It cannot even be said that one group is better than the other, or that either of these categories has any specific characteristics. **Therefore all we can do is increase the potency gradually and watch for the reaction, as this book is all about.**

Part Seven

ADDITIONS

Specifics of self-treatment

Technically, doing self-treatment is not different from treating someone else. Everyone who recommends autopathy to others has first tried it on himself or herself, and if not (only very hypothetically possible), they should have done so. A detailed knowledge of personally-experienced procedures would make it easier for us to understand what happens in other people. These would help us better orientate our own autopathic development: Setting apart the required time for self-examination, the initial one, as well as for the later follow-ups. We do not cheat ourselves.

Come to realize concrete goals, what we want to cure or improve in ourselves: the problems, diseases, attributes. **Write down the individual subjective and objective observations, symptoms and their details** (the initial examination, page 20).

We establish the optimal values of **the three parameters** (page 46) for ourselves and apply the AP.

We record the date of all the changes and differences from ordinary daily fluctuations of the condition. There might be feelings and observations that have both negative and positive significance (higher temperature, itching, tiredness, more energy, better sleep, improvement or departure of a pathological symptom, etc).

During regular follow-ups we return to the previous self-examinations and **compare the current state of every symptom against what we recorded in the past.** We do not do these follow-ups unnecessarily often.

We always ask ourselves if our case is developing in line with Hering's Laws, meaning if the symptoms are in the main improving (even slowly) **in the direction from within outward.** *If not, we* **do not change the set-up of the three parameters.**

We will not let ourselves be confused or rushed by short-term (a day-long, or several day-long) fluctuations of the condition. **If the effectiveness is reduced, we increase dilution/potency. We do the same if there is no effect.**

Even in self-treatment **let's not forget the rules of treatment.** Let's think about them, leaf through the book to remind ourselves.

If the **current method of preparation loses effectiveness,** and increasing the potency did not help, or if the characteristics of the case are changing, then we can move onto **another method,** which would be more in accordance with the current situation (page 33).

Missing perspective of the situation. For example, I have cured my headaches and the chronic back pains with the particular set-up of the treatment's three parameters, but now my knee hurts, which is an old problem that used to hurt me years ago. I could easily forget about the healed problems, but now I need to remind myself of them to realize that I should not change the set-up that had been working up to yesterday, and that had helped the problems departing from inside to out, or even bring about a problem-free state. I therefore decide *not to change the potency or the method of making preparation, but I can shorten the interval between applications.* If I did not include the already solved problems in my deliberations, and let myself be carried away by the urgency of the situation (for instance, I want to go on a skiing trip with friends tomorrow), I might begin to increase the potency, or even lower it, or change the method of preparation. Just because I read that somebody's knee problem was solved differently, I could easily get lost in these thoughts. The shortest way to healing the knee would therefore be repeating the potency and the method of preparation that has proven functional before.

In urgent cases we may shorten the interval between applications, perhaps even to once a day, or similar. Sometimes this has worked even with the higher potencies, such as 12–30 liters.

If we happen to be under the *"wait and watch"* system after a one-off application, and our problems were being solved in the direction "from inside to out", and these inner improvements (such as quality of sleep) are persisting, and then an old more surface-like problems appears (the old symptom reappearing), *the quickest way of its elimination would be to simply wait.*

With self-treatment it is good to have someone around who knows you, and happens to know something about autopathy as well (it does not have to be a trained consultant), who can remind you of things. For instance, if the hypothetically totally unacceptable situation with the sore knee – which prevents you from making the ski trip – has only been here since yesterday (when you were healthier than before), then it is therefore not necessary to panic just because of a ski trip and change the set-up of three parameters. When you are drowning in your current problem, and someone reminds you of this (it could even be this book), you say A-HA! You will not change anything. If the whole family uses autopathy (a quite common situation), or a friend, it would not be difficult to find such a person. Another possibility is visiting a consultant in autopathy.

Impatience and rashness could be bad advisors. *If in the process of autopathic development we do not know what to do in the given situation, often it is best not doing anything (autopathic). Maybe there is a healing crisis, and the next day it would be different. Such things have happened.*

As for the crisis and old symptoms reappearing, as well as any other health situations that life brings our way: **Always take into account the possibility of consulting with a medical practitioner.**

Courses and further education

The majority of the current users of autopathy have up to now made their first practical steps following the book *Get Well With Autopathy*. When at the beginning of a course I ask the participants, which ones have already had experience with autopathy, usually about a third to half of them would put up their hands. Some, during the course, talk about their experiences. Often it comes out that practicing only by the books can bring about great results.

Still, the courses are beneficial. The more information we have, the better we can make use of the experiences that others have had before us. Not everything can be contained in books. Sometimes we deal with special situations, exacting cases and similar things, of which as yet there was nothing in books. During courses we show videos of serious and incurable problems, and also the follow-ups, where we can see how the problems depart, in which order, how we select the three parameters of treatment in accordance to the collection of symptoms, age,

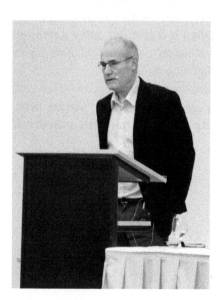

changeable situations, and how this happens in practice. During courses questions are being asked, and I answer them. The questions are usually informative and to the point.

Once when I was signing several dozens of **certificates of completion** of all three courses, I noticed that the percentage of those

The author at a conference.

graduating who had academic titles was close to 40%, significantly higher than the average in the population. I do not want to say that one needs a university degree to understand autopathy. Far from it – autopathy is based on simple principles, and the moment we accept them and learn how to use them, we become the experts. I would rather think that people who come to the courses do realize the practical value of education, who wish to attain the highest possible expertise – even in using the most precious thing we have, the life force, the reception of which is essential for maintaining our health. None of the participants apparently has any problem with the fact that here we deal with the fine-matter (from the materialistic point of view a non -material) information.

Autopathic courses II and III always follow several months after the previous one, and the participants gather practical experience during that time. In the second and third ones no one is without a personal experience.

In the second course we also go through cases of serious chronic states, such that – want it or not – nearly everyone would encounter within one's family and circle of friends, let

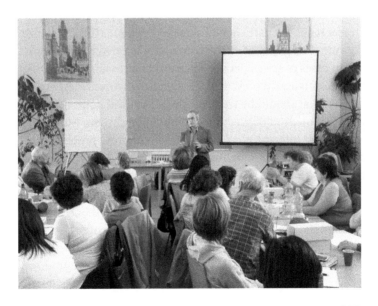

alone a consultancy practice. In the third, the subject matter is summarized, the participants' orientation in various techniques improves, there is more talk about high potencies, and more on the practical experiences.

To gain a certificate as a consultant in autopathy, with the possibility of having one's contact details published on the map of consultants at www.autopathy.com, currently a certificate is required from a **two-day practical seminar**, consisting of two Saturdays about three months apart. On the first meeting we jointly analyze six difficult cases, such as cases some participants could not solve or have been stuck with, and have brought their records of. We explain every step in analyzing and asking about the details. The participants themselves suggest the courses of action, which are discussed, with some being accepted and others rejected. Finally we make recommendations for the three parameters of treatment. Three months later we jointly went through all the cases and their records of development. And we found out that most of *the difficult cases that we have jointly analyzed have significantly improved, many problems have passed, and that the health of most of the people analyzed had been meaningfully improved. In some cases we corrected our recommendations and made some other more appropriate to their present state.* The participants firm their opinions that following the rules brings about success, and have learned how to apply this to cases of actual people. Such joint discussions of chronic cases, sometime in presence of the person involved, helps us to realize what should be treated, where the focal point of a case is, which method of preparation should be chosen, which potency, what interval, etc… The opinions of those present complement each other, sometimes even clashing in discussion and it appears to really confirm that more heads do know more.

Maybe it is an *inspiration for forming groups*, where people may gather, analyze, discuss, argue, and above all describe their recommendations to help someone, either present or not. It is, for example, possible for someone belonging to the group, to invite the person who is being treated that they do not know what to do with, but the common analyses can also be centered on individual members of the group, if they agree with it. And it works. There are no reasons against a few people making an agreement about meeting regularly twice a year. It is interesting, sometimes even suspenseful, never boring, and it helps the state of the participants' health, as well as their education. And a joint feeling of a job well done is also formed, working with the higher, fine-matter sphere of a person.

There are also **three-day spring seminars,** which have been held regularly for a number of years in a countryside hotel, where a couple of dozen people analyze the reports counselors or directly of chronically ill people speaking of their ordeals. The content is really the same, except that missing are the follow-up interviews, which are done by the consultant who had the particular person brought with them, or that person would continue in self-treatment, which has been done before. During the discussions and talks by the evening campfire one can often learn about autopathy more than at some lecture.

Important events are the day-long *Advanced Courses*, scheduled annually in fall. Autopathy is developing, and the people who attend are those who have been using autopathy for a long time (even ten, sixteen years), to find out about what is new, and what have we discovered in the process of our continuing practice.

For additional education there are also about hour-long *video lectures*, which are available on www.autopathy.com. One of them was to about a hundred listeners and it was titled *Autopathy and parasites.* Another lecture available on the Internet was held in a theatre in the historical center of Prague and its theme was *Autopathic self-treatment.*

I also conduct **webinars.** In 2016 there were three. Participants are mostly people who live too far and who practice autopathy by the books – some of them went through courses. There is always some main theme, which I deliver a short lecture about. People then ask questions via chat on various things, mainly regarding their own experiences and their cases of autopathy. They are visited by people from the USA, Canada, Switzerland, Germany, Hungary, Hong Kong, etc. Some of them have, after reading *Get Well With Autopathy* and participating in webinars, become professional consultants – mainly those who have also added autopathy to their existing practice as homeopaths, coaching of yoga, physiotherapy, Tchi-Kung, etc. Presently about five hundred trained consultants can be found on the map of consultants on www.autopathy.com. Some work in other European countries and in North America, or elsewhere. Some offer consultancy via Skype or over the telephone.

Autopathy is healing by water, and this has a cultural and historical context in the European *spa tradition*. Why not go to an autopathic spa, not only for the body, but also for the soul, for your prana, where we can meet with specialized consultants, who can express their opinion on our problems, who will in their lectures teach us how to treat ourselves or our near ones? I am only planning the first such *autopathic fitness camp*, though its already tested, and successful prototype are the Spring Seminars, with a verified wonderful atmosphere, when people visit nearby springs with an autopathy bottle, have discussions, educate themselves, and heal themselves.

Questions and answers

Question: Does the autopathy bottle have a parallel in history?

A long time ago, during their wanderings, Buddhist monks used to carry in a special pouch a vessel called a **kundika.** The Chinese traveler I Tsing writes about this in his book *Record of Buddhist Religion.* He travelled to India in the 7th century to study the habits and lifestyle of the monks, and to bring his report home, where Buddhism was still only beginning to take root. The vessel was made of fired clay. It was different from other vessels, having an opening on the round body, where water poured into the funnel from above could freely pour out. It was therefore a kind of flow-through device. I Tsing does not mention the purpose of the vessel in his book, and the contemporary exhibits in various museums do not offer any explanation either. The traveler only says that water in the kundika had to be clean and "untouched". The technique of using the bottle must have therefore been passed directly from the master to his pupil by word of mouth.

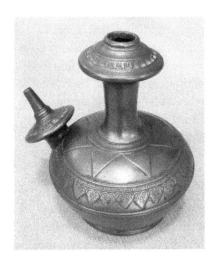

Decorative Chinese kundika from the 19th century. Its original ancient form and purpose were probably forgotten at that time. The funnel above is partially covered.

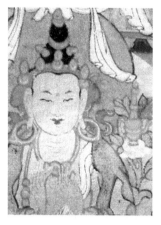

Maitreya, the anticipated Buddha of the next or rather upcoming age, usually depicted with a kundika by his left side. Here, the thangka in the Tibetan tradition, painted on canvas (detail). Maitreya is a principle, similarly Buddhahood is a principle, it does not have to relate to an actual person, it is latently present in every person. The energy of Maitreya principle is now felt by an increasing number of people. It would, according to prophecies, beccome manifested in the time of the highest materialism, when the spiritual dimension of people are being denyed, which could be just here and now.

Archaeologists have found hundreds of broken kundikas in ruins of extinct monasteries, mainly in their rubbish dumps, which means that kundika was not a ritual object used in worship, but rather an object of daily use. Kundikas were of various forms; in most of them it is possible to discern the funnel and the round vortex chamber with a draining pipe on the side. I noticed kundikas about two years after beginning to use the AB, and I was taken by the obvious similarity, as well as the use of "clean water that heals", as stated in the description of an old painting of Maitreya with a kundika. The word kundika has an obvious association with the word kundalini, so-called "serpent power", a concept known from yoga. Kundalini, similarly to prana, is associated with the fine energies that connect us to the Universe. A kundika was used to stimulate the fine information sphere and its connection to the physical body even in pre-Buddhist India. Preserved even is "Kundika upanishada", from between 4th and 8th century BC, where it is stated that the use of the kundika stimulates prana, increases vitality and the senses, strengthens the connection with the higher level of being (Brahman), and brings about strength and calmness.

Of course, the old kundikas with their shape would only produce low level informational potency, suitable to people of that era, who were far better tuned-up to the fine higher sphere, and in addition to that they ate only bio-food and breathed mostly clean air. To get that effect even nowadays, at the end of Kali Juga, the age of materialism, it is necessary to use high homeopathic potencies that can easily been made up in an autopathy bottle – a kundika of modern times.

In the old religions, advice and instructions on living a practical life were also given. When a monk walked through a countryside infested with malaria, he needed to have protection. A kundika would have certainly helped him in this. And when we walk through the contaminated country of today, we may also remember it.

A question: I am a rather intuitively founded person. What if I don't feel like reading this complicated book, keep any records, or be constantly bogged in some symptoms? Could I still use autopathy?

Yes. After all, I know of cases of people, who helped themselves very much, and who belonged exactly into this category. Some have even used a pendulum to determine the three parameters. The pendulum is actually an indicator of intuition. But you need to know how to use it. I have heard of failures, too.

Some people have taken it randomly, without reading books. And it worked from the beginning, even worked beautifully. Read about the case of self-treatment by Mrs Diana Becerova, put forward at the 8th conference: www.autopathy.com/I am grateful for joy.

She describes that she had an acute temperature and a years-long feeling of a life disaster. Somebody brought her a bottle and the book, which she did not read. However, instead she hastily made up an AP from saliva and 3 liters. The acute illness had improved even the same day. She repeated the application daily. "After about two weeks, I realized that I can feel happiness in my chest. A kind of feeling that I no longer remembered having. At first it surprised me, and I didn't know whether I should attribute it to autopathy or to same sort of happenstance. Nowadays I can safely say that autopathy made a miracle with my soul. The mental problems have improved by 90%. … I'm grateful for the feelings of joy that I can once again feel within myself. I remember that feeling well from my childhood, when I used to run in the meadow and was a fairy."

The simple method – how to not study autopathy, but still use it

I will give you a piece of advice on a very simple method of how not to read this book and not rack your brains over anything, and still use autopathy:

*Choose a basic **method of preparation from breath**, from instructions that are included in the box with the AB. Start with 1 liter of water. Apply daily. If something in your feelings begins to improve, keep repeating applications. If not, after a week increase to 1.5 liters (one bottle of water). If something in your feelings improves, keep applying, if not, after a week add another bottle with 1.5 liters of water … and so on. If you reach 6 liters, move onto the interval of once a week. If nothing improves, read this book from beginning to end.*

"Whichever" autopathy is better than no autopathy.

Acronyms

AB   autopathy bottle
AP   autopathic preparation
B   preparation from breath
BB   boiled breath
S   preparation from saliva
SB   saliva boiled
SBB   saliva mixed with breath, boiled
P1–P5   prana, preparation from information of the seventh chakra
UB   urine boiled

Examples of how to use already existing names of diseases and faults

The effect of autopathy could ever only be on the whole, **we act on the non-material life force, prana,** which organizes the body and the mind, and maintains harmony in the whole system. *Autopathy is not a device to battle against such-and-such disease.* Nonetheless, it is being used by people who have been given some diagnoses or test results. **It appears that for people of certain characteristics of problems, some types of AP could *in the beginning* be more suitable than others.** The state of life force is reflected in the state of our body and mind, and through this we determine the three parameters of autopathic effect. It is therefore necessary to take into account all other displays and characteristics of the given person that describe the wholeness and life satisfaction, not only the names of diseases, and always use up our entire *optimization technique.*

We do not form any diagnoses of our own. It is always about the overall assessment of the disruption of life force. The criterion of diagnoses and tests in autopathy could only be of additional, auxiliary value, and we can do without it. **We only take it into account when the given problem is being felt as "the focal point of the case", as being the most important.** When we know that the stated method of making preparation has worked with people having the same problem, we can use it.

Allergy – BB, HS, S, B, P5
Alopecia, excessive falling of hair in women – SB
Alzheimer's disease – S
Anorexia, bulimia – P5, B
Arthritis – BB
Asthma bronchial - BB
Autism – SB, B
Autoimmune diseases – BB
Cancer – alternating SBB and P5

Candida, yeast, discharges, coated tongue, inflammation of nail beds, hangnails – BB, SBB
Chlamydia pneumoniae and trachomatis – BB
Cirrhosis of liver – BB
Crohn's disease – alternating BB and BS
Depression, fear, anxiety – P2, P5, B
Diabetes – SB, BB, S
Eczema – SB, SBB
Finishing the treatment – B – higher potencies
Gout, high lever of uric acid in blood – UB
Gynecological inflammation – SB, SBB
Heart and vessel problems – BB
Hemorrhoids – BB
Influenza – SB, BB, P5
Infertility – BB, B, P5
Injury, first aid – S
Injury, long-term corollary – SB, BB, P5
Insomnia – S, P5, B
Intestine problems – BS
Liver tests, bad – BB
Lupus erythematosus – BB
Lyme disease - BB
Migraine – BB, S
Psoriasis – SB
Psychological stress, trauma – P2
Rheumatic problems – BB
Tinnitus – BB
Tonsillitis – SB
Toxoplasmosis – BB
Ulcerous colitis – SB, alternating BB and SB

Dictionary of terms

Here you will find a list and explanation of terms. Most of them are normally not taught at schools and used by media. You should note that majority of them have some connection to the systems of idealistic philosophy, or to the traditional systems of spirituality. This is so because the schools teach, the media stress and the state-supported philosophy (or religion) is materialism, which does not recognize the fine sphere of man, and does not offer any key to understanding or describing what is happening in autopathy.

At the age of thirty-three I discovered homeopathy and Buddhism, and the similarity of both these systems enthralled me. It was particularly the compatibility of their methods and concepts of the two, together with their common aim – relieving and freeing humankind from suffering. In relation to other people, there is then the essentiality and cultivation of the basic human instinct: compassion. Therefore, my terminology is not only influenced by homeopathy, but also by Buddhism, because this corresponds with my way of thinking. Nevertheless, I need to stress that **the autopathic principle of treatment is not tied to any philosophy**, religion or anything similar. It is simply here, and our knowledge of it, and how it works, and how we should use it, comes entirely from our experiences of observing of what happens after applying an aptly chosen preparation on humans, animals, and even plants. What we do is a practical, empirical way of using an up-till-recently unknown (or forgotten) universal principle of therapy. The aim of our practice is to ease or remove suffering in us or in other people. Faith itself is of no importance, as far as the result is concerned. No matter what you believe in, you desire health, which is not in conflict with any faith. Autopathy can help you. Not once have I seen autopathy improve the health of a skeptical materialist (a person who believes that he or she is made up entirely from matter and that his or her consciousness and mind is only a result of physical processes). Such persons, usually in the end, somehow manage to integrate autopathy with their system of belief, or at least set it aside under the label of "there are more things in heaven and earth…", or "science keeps developing, and it might one day discover the mechanism that is behind it". And this is fine. In fact, such a person is right. I believe – and again and again can see – that autopathy can fit into the life of a person of any philosophy, religion, or any conviction. As our experience shows us, the users of this practical method do not have any urgent need of putting it into any philosophical or religious frame.

Chakras – fine matter informational centers or channels, through which our body receives prana, Qi, life force, and is being formed. Over our seven personal chakras (diagram page 39) there are other, less personal chakras, the highest chakra of anyone is the universal Source. It belongs to all of us.

Death – the inevitable end of the body, which must come sooner or later to everybody. Departure from the physical body, which to the live and constantly developing mind ceased to be of any more help. The human mind endures, keeps changing, but does not perish.

Disease – a malfunction, disorder in harmony, fault in health, caused by the system of body and mind being out-of-tune towards the reception of creative vital information from the higher fine-matter (spiritual) organizational sphere.

Fine-matter – the word with a meaning close to "spiritual", is used in Buddhist tradition. It expresses well that the prototype of physical and mental processes is to be found in the fine sphere.

Incurable disease – a disorder in the harmony of the body and/ or mind, which cannot be repaired, usually because of personal karmic obstacles to treatment, given also for instance by age, unsuitable environment, structural changes in the organism, inappropriate lifestyle, addictions, wrong convictions, etc. Sometimes a disease might be there to teach the person something substantial, for instance how to change their attitude towards people, the world, one's own person, the Source... If the lesson is lost, the disease lasts. More rarely we might even see a disease that is there to prevent a person from their own self-destruction, by making it impossible for him or her to do things hurtful to themselves or to others. There is a vast scale of possibilities for karma to impede treatment, or to the contrary, to assist it.

Karma – *the summary of inner and outer factors, forming the present state of an individual, which have come into existence as a result of his or her thinking and actions, during the present life, or at other times.* The complexity of such causes is usually not known to people. The word was once used only in Brahmanic religions and Buddhism, and has now become common in the modern languages in Europe and America, even though it is sometimes incorrectly interpreted as an inevitability given by fate. Karma can be changed by conscious decision and appropriate actions of a given person. All actions of mind and body are either karmically beneficial or karmically harmful. *Prevalence of the second can cause autopathy to be limited.* Autopathy belongs among the karmically beneficial influences, because it reduces suffering. In Buddhist tradition there is the cycle of lives, during which karma could be changed and ripened to further stages of development. Such a universal karmic principle is being and was recognized in different philosophical and religious systems, including early Christianity.

Life force – prana, Qi – various names given by various cultures and therapeutic systems to the fine-matter stream of information that comes from the Universal Source. Through Yin and Yang, the binary code, it forms our mind and body, as well as the whole Universe, from its smallest to the largest parts, including our mind and body. Pythagoras had named these harmonic vibrations of the Universe, which create us and our world, "music of the spheres"; meanwhile Taoists call it Qi. The concept of life force has developed throughout the history of European natural healing, and is also used in homeopathy.

Matter – in idealistic teachings, including part of the contemporary science, it is perceived as one of the manifestations of consciousness, of mind. "The doctrine that the world is made up of objects whose existence is independent of human consciousness turns out to be in conflict with quantum mechanics and with facts established by experiment". Bernard d 'Espagnat, French quantum physicist.

Optimization – right from the beginning of autopathy being used, it was discovered that the mere unrefined saliva, diluted in an AB, can remove serious or even so-called incurable diseases. Subsequent developments have shown that there are limits beyond which the person in question cannot improve further, but other discovered methods of preparation from breath, saliva boiled and prana have been able to do it, after all. A similar one-off application sometimes helped a great deal, and sometimes not so well, but regular applications might have turned out to be in actual cases more effective, etc. We have gone through a journey on which we have collectively gathered a rich body of experiences, on the base of which the rules were laid down to make it possible for us to act optimally. This book is about the optimization of our use of autopathy.

Out-of-tune, being – a reduced ability to accurately accept prana, which comes from the Source. It can be caused, for instance, by external toxic influences, stress, etc. Health wanes in proportion to the degree of being out-of-tune, which manifests itself by growing chaos, disorder, disease, and suffering.

Potency – a traditional term in homeopathy, marking the degree of dilution, the amount of water poured through the AB.

Prana – see life force.

Relapse – reappearance of the original pathology after an already improved or cured state; the end of effectiveness of a particular AP.

Resonance – the vibrations of life force and the autopathic preparation are similar or almost the same, therefore a relationship between them is formed, which could make the body and mind sound once more through the influence of life force – the reception of which has improved.

The Source – the highest part of the Universe is the Source. In various times – including our current time, and in different parts of the world, it was given various philosophical or religious names. Plato called it the Idea. In China it is called Tao, in India Brahman, the Buddhists paint it on their pictures as the Avalokiteshvara (I have gone into more detail of this in *Get Well With Autopathy*, 6th edition), or it is called the Great Mind. In the Christian tradition it is for instance known as Swedenborg's Man, in the tradition of Christian science (in the USA influential system of healing) it is Christ. The Source has a fine-matter (spiritual) character, and "all that is" comes from it and is its parts. Including ourselves, humankind has in the Universe a central position. To what degree we are tuned-up to the Source determines how healthy we are.

Treatment, cure – in autopathy this means tuning-up the system of body and mind, its fine-matter information sections, to better receive the fine-matter information, known as prana, Qi, life force, which forms and organizes the individual mind and body.

Tuning-up – everything is frequencies, melodies, vibrations. Beginning with the structures of the body and mind, up to the elemental particles or galaxies. This is according to contemporary science, Taoists, Swedenborg, Buddhists, etc. We tune ourselves to the better reception of vibrational information, life force, prana, which function on the principle of Yin and Yang, binary code, information that forms us as a being, and which has a character of fine-matter. It emanates from one fine-matter Source, which is outside of space and time, being everywhere, in everything, which joins us all together, and which is our highest common chakra. We can liken ourselves to a radio playing pleasant music, which was subjected to strain when someone has knocked it down and thus put it out of tune. The radio is no longer resonating with the transmitter, it hums and cracks, the music is distorted, and the harmony is gone. We could however restore it by tuning-up the signal from the transmitter. The *resonance* – and therefore the harmony – comes back.

Untreatable case – a person karmically limited, as much as this.

Part Eight

THE INSTRUCTIONS FOR MAKING AN AUTOPATHIC PREPARATION

The common parts of all instructions for making an AP

All instructions for making different AP have the beginning and end parts in common. To save space, I only give them here, and the steps that follow on the next pages relate only to the actual making of the preparation.

At the beginning of the text:

AUTOPATHY BOTTLE – INSTRUCTION FOR USING

Read carefully before making the preparation.
Never take the bottle out of its plastic wrapper before commencing work on a preparation. The making of a preparation usually involves the person to whom the preparation would be applied, but this is not necessarily the case. The person making the preparation must be an adult.

The purpose: "The bottle" is so designed that by gradually flowing water through, it dilutes the information contained in one's own breath (or saliva, etc…), moving it to a fine-matter level (from the materialistic point of view, non-material). The product of the dilution is used exclusively by the person from whom the breath, saliva (etc…) originates.

Philosophy: On the basis of resonance, the product of a high level dilution has beneficial effects on the spiritual, fine-matter (or from the materialistic point of view, *non-material*) organizational system in a person, known also as "life-force", the "prana", or "Qi".

(Here belongs the practical instruction related to each specific kind of preparation. Please see the following pages for these steps.)

At the end of the text:

Due to the "memory of glass", the fine-matter information remains in the material of the bottle even after the liquid has been removed. For this reason **the autopathic bottle can be used for one person only.** Experience has shown that with repeated applications, **the bottle must be changed for a new one three months after its first use,** otherwise the influence of the "memory of glass" will result in the loss of effect.

The bottle is to be returned immediately after use to its plastic wrapper that does not need to be sealed any more, and put into its box, so that there is no contamination (spoilage) caused by another person touching it, or breathing on it , passing droplets while talking, etc. Bottles no longer in use should not be kept, but should go into sorted waste disposal.

From 1 liter of water, a dilution of 40 C is made.

It is helpful, though not essential, to use the advice of a trained consultant. The development of one's condition after applying the preparation might not be simple; it is individual – dependent on the inner, hidden, karmic state of the person.

The use of the thus made preparation is not a substitute for medical care. It is not intended to diagnose, treat, mitigate, cure or prevent any disease.

The device is RCD protected. It is not a medicinal device.

Complete instructions are also available on www.autopathy. com/instructions, where they can be downloaded and printed. Videos of preparations being made are also there.

Preparation made of boiled breath

Requirements:
1. "Autopathy bottle" made of laboratory glass.
2. The amount of water recommended by a consultant or literature (minimum of 1 liter); spring water in plastic bottles (without a high content of minerals, without any additives and not sparkling), or clean bottled distilled water.
3. A gas burner, portable gas burner, or camping gas burner.

Procedure:
1. For at least an hour before do not eat, drink, put anything into your mouth, or make cell phone calls.
2. If we make the preparation for someone else, then cover your mouth and nose with a scarf or face mask before unwrapping the AB, so that any droplets of saliva or breath (while sneezing, talking, breathing from up close, etc.) will not be transmitted into the preparation. No other person should be present.
3. Unwrap the bottle and hold it in hand so that both pipes leading from the circular vortex chamber are up at the angle of 45 degrees, in the shape of the letter V. Pour into the bottle a small amount of diluting water, to completely fill the round vortex chamber at the bottom of the bottle. The level of water should be about 1.5cm/0.6" into both pipes. Do not touch the inside of the bottle.
4. After taking a deep breath, put one nostril to the end of the shorter tube, while holding/blocking the other nostril, and with a long, slow out breath, blow air bubbles into the water in the chamber. Repeat with the other nostril. Immediately heat up the contents of the round chamber, until the water boils. Touch the lower part of the round chamber with the flame. Hold the bottle with a folded napkin, as it will be hot. Do not aim the tubes towards yourself or any other people, as there is a danger

of splashing hot water. After the water begins to boil, let it boil for about 30 seconds. Then put the bottle on the edge of a hand basin (or hold it there with your hand), with the drainage tube towards the drain. About 30 seconds later steadily begin to pour the amount of water recommended by a consultant or literature through the funnel. Pour from the height of about 5cm/2". Do not touch the funnel. Throughout the diluting process the water in the funnel should level up. If it overflows, it does not matter.

5. Immediately after this pour the contents of the round chamber of the bottle or its part (a few drops would suffice) through the lower tube to the center of the forehead, and spread it downwards with a light touch of the lower tube, above the root of the nose, in the area of the sixth chakra. Allow the skin to dry.

Preparation made of saliva boiled

Requirements:
1. "Autopathy bottle" made of laboratory glass.
2. The amount of water recommended by a consultant or literature (minimum of 1 liter); spring water in plastic bottles (without a high content of minerals, without any additives and not sparkling), or clean bottled distilled water.
3. In the case of a person who cannot spit, an unused sterile dropper.
4. A gas burner, portable gas burner, or camping gas burner.

Procedure:
1. The evening before making the preparation we clean our mouth. First thing in the morning we spit into the autopathy bottle. Before that we cough several times with the closed lips, so that the droplets from the respiratory system get into the mouth. Before this we do not eat, drink, or put anything into your mouth, or make cell phone calls. There should not be any cosmetic products on the face or the lips.
2. Do not touch the inside of the funnel. No other person should be present. If we make the preparation for someone else, we have our mouth and nose covered with a scarf or surgical mask throughout the preparation process. Spit a small amount of saliva to the funnel. In the case of a person who cannot spit, take the saliva from their mouth with a dropper (one drop is enough).
3. Hold the bottle in hand so that both pipes leading from the round vortex chamber are up at the angle of 45 degrees, in the shape of the letter V. We wash the small amount of saliva down with a small amount of diluting water to the round vortex chamber at the bottom of the bottle. Immediately heat up the contents of the round chamber, until the water boils. Touch the lower part of

the round chamber with the flame. Hold the bottle with a folded napkin, as it will be hot. Do not aim the tubes towards yourself or any other people, as there is a danger of splashing hot water. After the water begins to boil, keep boiling for about 30 seconds. Wait about 30 seconds. Then put the bottle on the edge of a hand basin (or hold it there with our hand), with the drainage tube towards the drain.

4. Steadily pour the amount of water recommended by a consultant or literature through the funnel. Pour from the height of about 5cm/2". Throughout the diluting process the water in funnel should level up. If it overflows, it does not matter.

5. Immediately after this pour the contents of the round chamber of the bottle or its part (a few drops would suffice) through the lower tube to the center of the forehead, and spread it downwards with a light touch of the lower tube, above the root of the nose, in the area of the sixth chakra. Allow the skin to dry.

Preparation from breath

Requirements:

1. "Autopathy bottle" made of laboratory glass.
2. The amount of water recommended by a consultant or literature (minimum of 1 liter); spring water in plastic bottles (without a high content of minerals, without any additives and not sparkling), or clean bottled distilled water.

The Procedure:

1. At least for an hour beforehand do not eat, drink, or put anything into your mouth, or make cell phone calls.
2. Unwrap the bottle and hold it in hand so that both pipes leading from the circular vortex chamber are up at the angle of 45 degrees, in the shape of the letter V. Pour a small amount of diluting water into the bottle, to completely fill the round vortex chamber at the bottom of the bottle. The level of water should be about 1.5cm/0.6" into both pipes. Do not touch the inside of the funnel.
3. After taking a deep breath, put the end of the shorter tube to one nostril, while holding/blocking the other nostril, and with a long, slow out breath make air bubbles through the water in the chamber. Repeat with the other nostril. In the vortex chamber there will be a small amount of water carrying the information. Then put the bottle on the edge of a hand basin (or hold it there with your hand), with the drainage tube towards the drain.
4. Immediately after this begin to steadily pour the amount of water recommended by a consultant or literature through the funnel. Pour from the height of about 5cm/2", and do not touch the funnel. Throughout the diluting process the water in the funnel should level up. If it overflows, it does not matter.
5. Instantaneously after this pour the contents (or part of

its contents – a few drops would suffice) of the round chamber of the bottle to the center of the forehead, and spread it there with a light touch of the lower tube, above the root of the nose in the area of the sixth chakra. Allow the skin to dry.

Preparation from saliva

Requirements:
1. "Autopathy bottle" made of laboratory glass.
2. The amount of water recommended by a consultant or literature (minimum of 1 liter); spring water in plastic bottles (without a high content of minerals, without any additives and not sparkling), or clean bottled distilled water.
3. In the case of a person who cannot spit, an unused sterile dropper.

The procedure:
1. Carefully clean your teeth with a brush without using any toothpaste. For at least half an hour beforehand do not eat, put anything into your mouth, or make cell phone calls. There should not be any cosmetic products on the face or lips.
2. If we make the preparation for someone else, we have our mouth and nose covered with a scarf or surgical mask throughout the preparation process when we take the saliva, so that no droplets of saliva or breath (while sneezing, talking, breathing from close up, etc.) are transmitted into the preparation. In the case of a person who cannot spit, take the saliva from their mouth with a dropper (one drop is enough).
3. Unwrap the bottle and stand it on the edge of a hand basin, or the bottom of it, with the bottom short tube aimed towards the drain. Or you can hold it in your hand. Do not touch the inner wall of the funnel. No other person should be present.
4. First spit away from the AB, then gather enough saliva in your mouth, and spit into the funnel. A small amount of saliva is enough, so long as it is visible. Wash the saliva into the round vortex chamber. Immediately after this begin to steadily pour the amount of water recommended by a consultant or literature through the funnel.

Pour from the height of about 5cm/2", and do not touch the funnel. Throughout the diluting process the water in funnel should level up. If it overflows, it does not matter.

5. Instantaneously after this pour the contents (or part of its contents – a few drops would suffice) though of the round chamber of the bottle to the center of the forehead, and spread it there with a light touch of the lower tube, above the root of the nose in the area of the sixth chakra. Allow the skin to dry.

The auto-nosode

Requirements and the beginning part of instruction (p. 221) are the same as for preparation from Saliva boiled (p. 225).

Procedure:
To make an auto-nosode from one's own stool, let a small piece of stool soak in water, which you have poured into a plastic lid from a bottle containing spring water. Let it wash in there with a round movement of the lid. Then with a sterile dropper take one drop of this water and put onto the inner wall of the AB's funnel. *From this moment continue (without spitting) according to the instructions for saliva boiled. The AP made from stool, urine etc. is meant for the person whose material was used.*

Prana 2

Requirements:
1. "Autopathy bottle" made of laboratory glass.
2. The amount of water recommended by a consultant or literature (minimum of 1 liter); spring water in plastic bottles (without a high content of minerals, without any additives and not sparkling), or clean bottled distilled water.
3. A surgical mask or scarf to cover the nose and mouth.

Procedure:
1. An hour before making the preparation do not make cell phone calls, and there must not be any cosmetic products on the face. No matter whom we make the preparation for – ourselves or someone else, have a scarf, napkin or surgical mask over the mouth before taking the bottle out of its wrapper. No other person should be present.
2. Unwrap the bottle, do not touch the inside of the funnel. Fill the round chamber at the bottom about a half full with water used for diluting. The tilted bottle is held near the funnel. Both pipes leading from the circular vortex chamber are up at the angle of 45 degrees, in the shape of the letter V.
3. The vortex chamber with a little water should be held over the head, roughly in line with the axis of the body, about 15-25cm/6-10" above the center of the head. The arm holding the bottle is slightly bent. Nothing needs to be measured; all is just estimated and approximate. At this level is our seventh chakra, which is not a point, but a spatial area.
4. First make a round, circular movement with the vortex chamber and water inside, move it up and down, then hold the vortex chamber still in the middle, in axis of the body, for about two minutes.

5. Standing next on the edge of a hand basin, pour the amount of water that was recommended by a consultant or by literature into the autopathy bottle. The water would level up in the funnel. If you spill some, that does not matter. Pour water from about 5cm/2" above the funnel.

6. With a part of the water from the bottle, moisten the middle of your forehead above the root of the nose, in the area of the sixth chakra. A few drops is enough, spread it there with the light movement of the pipe. Immediately after moistening the forehead, move the bottle with the rest of the water again above the head, into the area of the seventh chakra, where it was before, and leave it there for about half a minute. After this hold the round chamber with water for half a minute close to the forehead, in the area of the sixth chakra.

7. For the future use, put the bottle into the plastic wrapper and into the box, which you close. Take off the surgical mask or scarf.

Prana 5

Requirements:

"Autopathy bottle" made of laboratory glass.

The amount of water recommended by a consultant or literature (minimum of 1 liter); spring water in plastic bottles (without a high content of minerals, without any additives and not sparkling), or clean bottled distilled water.

A surgical mask or scarf to cover the nose and mouth.

Procedure:

An hour before making the preparation do not make cell phone calls, and there must not be any cosmetic products on the face. No matter whom we make the preparation for – ourselves or someone else, have a scarf, napkin or surgical mask over the mouth before taking the bottle out of its wrapper. No other person should be present.

Unwrap the bottle, do not touch the inside of the funnel. Fill the round chamber at the bottom about a half full with water used for diluting. The tilted bottle is held near the funnel. Both pipes leading from the circular vortex chamber are up at the angle of 45 degrees, in the shape of the letter V.

The vortex chamber with a little water should be held over the head, roughly in line with the axis of the body, about 15-25cm/6–10" above the center of the head. The arm holding the bottle is slightly bent. Nothing needs to be measured; all is just estimated and approximate. At this level is our seventh chakra, which is not a point, but a spatial area.

First make a round, circular movement with the vortex chamber and water inside, move it up and down, then hold the vortex chamber still in the middle, in axis of the body, for about two minutes.

Standing next on the edge of a hand basin, pour the amount of water that was recommended by a consultant or by literature into the autopathy bottle. The water would level up in the funnel. If you spill some, that does not matter. Pour water from about 5cm/2" above the funnel.

After this hold the bottle with the rest of the water in the round chamber in the area of each chakra, as described further:

With the diluting finished, hold the bottle with the rest of water slightly tilted backwards, so as not to spill it, back above the head, into the area of seventh chakra (scheme of the chakras on page 39), where it was before. Move it slightly up and down.

Hold for about 30 seconds. The same time applies also to the administration to each lower chakra. Then move the chamber with the water to within 1–2cm/0.4–0.8" away from the skin to the forehead, between the eyebrows, without touching (if that happens, it is no problem), with a slight movement within the space.

After this we hold the bottle for about the same time and in same distance from the throat chakra (Adam's apple, center of throat), then the heart (between the breasts), then solar plexus (2cm/0.8" above the navel), the second chakra (in front of the upper rim of pubic bone, between crotch and umbilicus). After this we hold the tilted bottle with the rest of the water in the space between both legs, under crotch, in the axis of the body, where the first chakra aiming towards the earth is situated, without touching.

After this hold the bottle in front of each chakra in the ascending order, up to the sixth chakra. This is where the application ends.

For further use put the bottle into the plastic wrapper and into the box, which you close. Take off the surgical mask or scarf.[1]

---

[1] Conversion table – liters to US fluid ounces to US gallons
1 L = 33.81 fl oz = 0.26 gal
1.5 L = 50.72 fl oz = 0.39 gal
For the purpose of autopathic preparation the conversion from liters can be rounded by 0.9 fl oz.
In cases of a preparation with carbon filter or by a spring, 1 minute of water flowing into the AB allows approximately 2 liters to go through, making the potency of 80 C.